An Introduction to Medical Teaching

Kathryn N. Huggett • William B. Jeffries

Editors

An Introduction to Medical Teaching

Second Edition

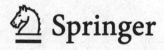
Springer

Editors
Kathryn N. Huggett
Office of Medical Education
Creighton University School of Medicine
Omaha, Nebraska, USA

William B. Jeffries
Office of Medical Education
University of Vermont College of Medicine
Burlington, Vermont, USA

ISBN 978-94-017-7786-5   ISBN 978-94-017-9066-6 (eBook)
DOI 10.1007/978-94-017-9066-6
Springer Dordrecht Heidelberg New York London

Printed on acid-free paper

Springer is part of Springer Science+Business Media (www.springer.com)

Preface

This book was conceived as a tool for the many varieties of medical teacher: the basic scientist, the clinical faculty member, the resident physician and the community practitioner. Individuals from each of these groups often assume the responsibility for educating the physicians of tomorrow. However, the formal training of these teachers is usually not centered on educational principles. Medical teachers often enter their careers ill equipped to engage in a scholarly approach to teaching. Thus we chose to create this volume as a how-to guide for medical teachers who wish to gain an understanding of educational principles and apply them to their teaching.

In keeping with the spirit of the book as an introduction, we have not produced a comprehensive textbook on medical education. Rather, the book is intended to introduce the reader to a variety of major topics that might serve specific needs. This work will be particularly useful to the educator who wants to introduce new methods into their teaching. As such, all of the chapters are grounded in the modern literature underlying adult learning theory and educational methods; however, the advice contained in each chapter is overwhelmingly practical and can be put to immediate use. The chapters begin with a focus on the learner, followed by a survey of the most common teaching modalities encountered by a medical teacher (large group, small group, problem-based, team based, clinical, simulation, and laboratory). We also examine critical elements that comprise the essentials of teaching and learning (using technology, student assessment, teaching evaluation, course design). Finally, we introduce the topic of educational scholarship and supply advice on documenting teaching for career advancement. In addition, to encourage the reader to further investigate each topic, chapters are fully referenced and the appendix provides additional educational resources.

The scope of educational scholarship is now quite broad. Thus no single author could adequately address the topics presented herein. We have thus assembled an exceptionally qualified and highly regarded team of authors who represent a diverse pool of teachers, clinicians and educational scholars. We are extremely grateful to the authors, who generously devoted their time and talents to this project.

Omaha, NE, USA   Kathryn N. Huggett
Burlington, VT, USA   William B. Jeffries

Contents

Contributors

Mark A. Albanese Professor Emeritus, Departments of Population Health Sciences and Educational Psychology, School of Medicine and Public Health and College of Education, University of Wisconsin-Madison, Madison, WI, USA

Azzam S. Al-Kadi Unaizah College of Medicine, Qassim University, Qassim, Saudi Arabia

M. Brownell Anderson Senior Academic Officer, International Programs, National Board of Medical Examiners, Philadelphia, PA, USA

Karen J. Brasel Department of Surgery-Trauma, Critical Care, Medical College of Wisconsin, Milwaukee, WI, USA

David Chia Yale Internal Medicine Primary Care Residency Program, New Haven, CT, USA

David A. Cook Division of General Internal Medicine, Mayo Clinic College of Medicine, Rochester, MN, USA

Laura C. Dast School of Medicine and Public Health, University of Wisconsin, Madison, WI, USA

Peter G.M. de Jong Leiden University Medical Center, Leiden, The Netherlands

Kristi J. Ferguson Carver College of Medicine, University of Iowa, Iowa City, IA, USA

Melissa A. Fischer University of Massachusetts School of Medicine, Worcester, MA, USA

Aviad Haramati Georgetown University Medical Center, Washington, DC, USA

Kathryn N. Huggett Office of Medical Education, Creighton University School of Medicine, Omaha, NE, USA

William B. Jeffries Office of Medical Education, University of Vermont College of Medicine, Burlington, VT, USA

N. Kevin Krane Tulane University School of Medicine, New Orleans, LA, USA

Brian Mavis OMERAD (Office of Medical Education Research and Development), Michigan State University College of Human Medicine, East Lansing, MI, USA

Cate Nicholas Clinical Simulation Laboratory, Fletcher Allen Health Care/ University of Vermont, College of Medicine, Burlington, VT, USA

Dean X. Parmelee Boonschoft School of Medicine, Wright State University, Dayton, OH, USA

Susan J. Pasquale Johnson and Wales University, Providence, RI, USA

Michele P. Pugnaire University of Massachusetts Medical School, Worcester, MA, USA

Janet M. Riddle Department of Medical Education, University of Illinois-Chicago College of Medicine, Chicago, IL, USA

Nicole K. Roberts The Academy for Scholarship in Education, Department of Medical Education, Southern Illinois University School of Medicine, Springfield, IL, USA

Majid Sadigh Danbury Hospital/Western Connecticut Health Center, University of Vermont College of Medicine, Burlington, VT, USA

Katrin Sara Sadigh Yale Internal Medicine Primary Care Residency Program, New Haven, CT, USA

Deborah Simpson Department of Family Medicine at UWSMPH & MCW, Academic Affairs – Aurora Health Care, Aurora UW Medical Group/Academic Administration, Milwaukee, WI, USA

Carole S. Vetter Department of Orthopedics, Medical College of Wisconsin, Milwaukee, WI, USA

Travis P. Webb Department of Surgery-Trauma, Critical Care, Medical College of Wisconsin, Milwaukee, WI, USA

List of Figures

List of Tables

Chapter 1
Facilitating Student Learning

Kristi J. Ferguson

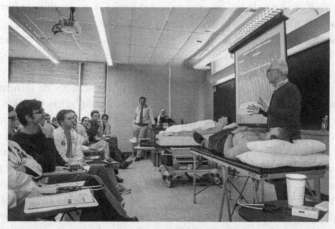

Abstract Helping students learn in medical education presents unique challenges that have changed rapidly over the last 10 years. For example, the growth of medical knowledge is accelerating exponentially, making it impossible for prospective physicians to learn everything they need to know during medical school, and making it essential for them to learn the skills related to lifelong learning that will serve them for their entire medical careers. Prospective physicians must learn how to identify their own learning needs, identify appropriate sources for addressing those needs, and learn how to apply the information and skills acquired to the care of patients during medical school and beyond. In addition, traditional models that feature pre-clinical training followed by 2 years of clinical training are giving way to newer models, which emphasize early application of basic science knowledge to clinical problems (e.g., through problem-based learning), as well as revisiting basic science content in the clinical years.

K.J. Ferguson, MSW, Ph.D. (✉)
Carver College of Medicine, University of Iowa,
Iowa City, IA 52242, USA
e-mail: kristi-ferguson@uiowa.edu

K.N. Huggett and W.B. Jeffries (eds.), *An Introduction to Medical Teaching*,
DOI 10.1007/978-94-017-9066-6_1, © Springer Science+Business Media Dordrecht 2014

Introduction

Helping students learn in medical education presents unique challenges that have changed rapidly over the last 10 years. For example, the growth of medical knowledge is accelerating exponentially, making it impossible for prospective physicians to learn everything they need to know during medical school, and making it essential for them to learn the skills related to lifelong learning that will serve them for their entire medical careers. Prospective physicians must learn how to identify their own learning needs, identify appropriate sources for addressing those needs, and learn how to apply the information and skills acquired to the care of patients during medical school and beyond. In addition, traditional models that feature pre-clinical training followed by 2 years of clinical training are giving way to newer models, which emphasize early application of basic science knowledge to clinical problems (e.g., through problem-based learning), as well as revisiting basic science content in the clinical years.

While growth in knowledge creates the need for lifelong learning, characteristics of students and their access to technology have changed as well. For example, incoming students have grown up with access to technology, and are accustomed to using it in their daily lives. This creates advantages as well as challenges for the medical educator. Using technology to store information for later retrieval is easy; being critical of available information and identifying sources of information that are valid is more difficult. Newer high-fidelity simulation allows students to learn and practice skills before they use them on patients, it provides opportunities for learning to work in teams to solve critical problems without putting patients at risk, and it provides a mechanism for assessing these skills in an authentic setting.

Later chapters in this book will address specific educational methods, e.g., Chap. 2 looks at the use of large group teaching methods, Chap. 3 addresses the use of small groups, Chap. 5 looks at problem-based learning, and Chap. 8 looks at simulation. Others will address issues of concern to the field in general, such as assessment of students, evaluation of teaching and learning, scholarship, and planning.

This chapter will begin with a discussion of key concepts related to helping students learn. It will then cover student-centered approaches, such as self-directed learning, that can enhance learning with understanding. Next, it will review the role of the teacher in developing appropriate learning activities and assessment strategies, and will conclude with a discussion of the role of feedback and the learning environment in enhancing student learning.

Key Terms

Active learning refers to instructional approaches that require learners to interact with the material in some fashion, as opposed to being passive recipients of information.

Self-directed learning means that learners control the objectives as well as the approach to their learning. It can also refer to control over the methods used to assess learning. Self-directed learning is more a matter of degree than an all-or-nothing proposition.

Surface learning refers to acquiring knowledge through memorization, without reflecting on it, and the main purpose of surface learning is often to meet external requirements.

Deep learning, on the other hand, relates prior knowledge to new information, integrates information across courses, and organizes content into a coherent knowledge base. Motivation for deep learning is more internal (to the student).

Scaffolding refers to assistance that students receive early on in their learning that is gradually taken away as students become more responsible for their own learning.

Learning environment in this chapter refers to the extent to which the overall organization of learning and support services demonstrates concern for students' well-being as well as for their academic achievement. The **hidden curriculum** refers to learning that occurs outside the classroom, and in medical education often refers to behavior observed by learners that demonstrates such attributes as honesty, respect, and professional values (or their absence).

Role of Learners

Marchese (1998) discusses several criteria that are associated with long-term learning and retention (see Table 1.1). Independent learning, having choices about what to learn, and building on students' intrinsic motivation and natural curiosity all present special challenges for medical educators. External forces such as accrediting bodies and licensing boards have a significant impact on the context of what medical students have to learn. Even so, it is possible to build more self-directed, motivating ways of learning into the curriculum. For example, one of the major benefits of problem-based learning is that students enjoy learning and spend more of their time in independent, self-directed learning. Team-based learning, which builds small group learning activities into large classes, may offer some of the benefits of problem-based learning within a more traditional structure. In addition, hybrid curricula that incorporate self-directed, small group learning experiences alongside traditional classes may offer some of the benefits of problem-based learning while maintaining some of the efficiency of large group teaching.

No matter what strategy is used, it is important to maintain students' natural curiosity about how the human body works and about how to take care of patients. Most students come to medical school with high levels of curiosity, but the more they are required to memorize isolated facts or engage in very deep learning about relatively esoteric principles, the less likely they are to maintain that enthusiasm. The challenge comes in identifying core material and teaching it in an interesting, clinically relevant manner.

Another aspect of the role of the learner concerns individual learning style. While learning style has been studied extensively, claims have been made based on minimal evidence in terms of the effect of learning style on learning outcomes, or of designing instruction to match an individual's learning style. That being said, there is little harm in designing instruction that has the potential to meet the needs of

Table 1.1 Criteria associated with long-term learning and retention

Role of the learner
Learners function independently
Learners have choices about what to learn and how to learn
Learners have opportunities to build on intrinsic motivation and natural curiosity
Role of the learning activities
Learning activities require the application of higher-order thinking skills
Learning activities mirror the tasks that learners will face in the real world
Role of feedback and assessment
Learners are able to practice and receive feedback in challenging interactions with other learners, with minimal threat
Learners receive frequent feedback and are encouraged to reflect on the feedback
Learners are assessed in ways that mirror the above criteria

Adapted from Marchese (1998)

students with varying learning styles. A traditional method to reinforce material in multiple ways is to offer instruction that students can both see and hear. For example, a lecture with slides and accompanying written materials reinforces the material in multiple ways. Other variants of learning style indicate whether the learner prefers to learn alone or with others. Since medical practice often involves interacting with other professionals as well as with patients, having practice interacting with colleagues in a learning environment is important even if an individual student's general preference is to work alone.

Role of the Teacher

How students learn is affected by how teachers teach. A model presented by Kern et al. (1998) and others is especially helpful in looking at the process of developing curriculum in medical education (see Fig. 1.1). Kern and colleagues talk about the importance of first doing a needs assessment, to determine what learners already know and what they need to know. Then the teacher must develop goals and objectives for learners. Once this process is complete, educators must develop strategies that will be effective in reaching those goals and objectives. Finally, the teacher must assess learners in ways that reflect the goals, objectives, and strategies.

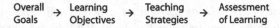

Fig. 1.1 Aligning goals, objectives, strategies, and assessment

Writing Objectives, Developing Strategies, and Designing Assessment Plans

In medical education, decisions about curriculum content are often made without first determining the overall goals and learning objectives. Goals are statements about the overall purposes of a curriculum. Objectives must be specific and measurable, and can be related to the learner, the process, or the outcomes of education. Each must be written in a way that allows for measurement to determine whether the objective has been achieved. Then strategies must be selected that allow the learner to achieve the desired objectives. Once the curriculum has been implemented, learners and the curriculum are evaluated, feedback is provided, and the cycle continues. Too often, educators select a teaching strategy without a clear idea of what they are trying to accomplish, e.g., incorporating small group teaching methods without understanding what such methods can reasonably accomplish or when they can be used most effectively.

Kern et al., discuss five types of objectives, each of which is most appropriately addressed by different types of educational strategies. For example, cognitive objectives related to knowledge acquisition can be taught by readings and lectures, while problem solving can be learned through problem-solving exercises or learning projects. Affective objectives may be achieved most appropriately through discussion, psychomotor skills must be demonstrated and practiced, while behavioral objectives may require real life experiences to be achieved.

Role of Learning Activities

Learning with understanding, as described in "How People Learn" (2000), assumes that a strong knowledge base of facts is important, but not sufficient for learning. Knowledge must be organized around important concepts, which improves understanding and ability to apply the knowledge to other contexts. Obtaining a large knowledge base involves being exposed to multiple examples of a given concept, active processing of the information, and use of higher-order thinking skills in working with the facts. Bloom's Taxonomy has been cited widely in educational circles. An approach that may be even more useful in medical education is Quellmalz' Taxonomy (see Table 1.2). The five levels are **Recall**, **Analysis**, **Comparison**, **Inference** and **Evaluation**.

At the **Recall** level, students remember key facts, and are asked to repeat them, either verbatim or by paraphrase. At the **Analysis** level, students break down a concept into separate components, and may look at cause/effect relationships. At the **Comparison** level, students are required to explain similarities and differences. At the **Inference** level, students may be given a generalization and asked to explain it, or they may be given the evidence and be asked to come up with a generalization. At the **Evaluation** level, students are asked to judge the worth of a particular statement or idea.

In order to encourage higher-order thinking, the goal should be to identify objectives, design teaching strategies, and assess learners at levels that are deeper

Table 1.2 Taxonomy of thinking skills

Category	Description	Sample questions and tasks
Recall	Remembering or recognizing key facts, definitions, concepts	Define the word digestion
	Repeating verbatim or paraphrasing information that has already been provided to the student	List the vital signs What is a normal blood pressure? Name the amino acids
Analysis	Understanding relationships between the whole and its component parts and between cause and effect	In what sequence did the symptoms occur?
	Sorting and categorizing	How does a blood pressure cuff work?
	Understanding how things work and how the parts of something fit together	Use the values provided to determine whether the patient is acidotic
	Understanding causal relationships	
	Getting information from charts, graphs, diagrams, and maps	
	Reflectively structuring knowledge in new ways	
Comparison	Explaining how things are similar and how they are different	In what ways are pneumonia and asthma alike?
	Comparisons may be either simple or complex	In what ways do they differ?
	Simple comparisons are based on a small number of very obvious attributes	Compare the risks and benefits to treatment of these
	Complex comparisons require an examination of a more sensitive set of attributes of two or more things	
	Comparisons start with the whole/part relationships in the analysis category and carry them a step further	
Inference	Reasoning inductively or deductively	What would happen if the patient lost 30 pounds?
	In deductive tasks, students reason from generalizations to specific instances and are asked to recognize or explain the evidence	Predict what will be the result if you stopped the patient's blood pressure medication
	In inductive tasks, students are given the evidence or details and are required to relate and integrate the information to come up with the generalization	Based on your research, what can you conclude about the need for this biopsy?
Evaluation	Expressing and defending an opinion	Is the experiment designed so that you will be able to tell whether the treatment is more effective than placebo?
	Evaluation tasks require students to judge quality, credibility, worth, or practicality using established criteria and explain how the criteria are met or not met	What is the most cost-effective way to diagnose pulmonary embolisms?

Adapted from Stiggins et al. (1988)

than simple recall of information. While learners need to have certain basic facts, it is in analyzing, comparing, drawing inferences, and evaluating information that learning for understanding occurs.

Requiring students to apply and integrate material may also require faculty members and course directors to integrate material across courses as well as across years of the curriculum. This means that faculty members need to know what is being taught in other courses, and, as much as possible, to reinforce learning that is going on in other courses. In a hybrid curriculum, this would mean that cases for problem based learning sessions are identified and selected based on the cases' ability to provide clinical relevance for what is being learned in the basic sciences, and for integrating material across courses.

Role of Feedback and Assessment

Another criterion identified by Marchese (1998) i.e., giving learners frequent feedback and encouraging them to reflect on the feedback, can be challenging in medical education as well. For example, evidence about the accuracy of learners' self-assessment suggests that higher achieving students tend to underestimate their performance while lower achieving students tend to over-estimate their performance. This makes the role of feedback and mentoring especially critical in helping students improve.

In the pre-clinical curriculum, too often the only form of feedback is exam scores, which may not allow sufficient time for students to reflect on exam performance and learn from their mistakes. The focus for reflecting on individual and class performance should be to identify areas of misunderstanding, and to identify ways in which the teaching or preparing for exams can be improved. Methods of assessment and feedback have powerful effects on student motivation. Giving students multiple chances for practice and feedback, for everything from interviewing skills and professional communication to knowledge about anatomy, can go a long way toward enhancing student learning. Doing so with groups of learners, so they can learn from each other, can be especially valuable, as long as the opportunities for practice and feedback occur in an environment supportive of learning and of the students. The key is to be sure that the assessment methods reward higher-order thinking skills.

Following are examples of general goals, learning objectives related to the goals, learning strategies appropriate for achieving the objectives, and methods for evaluating both learners and the process to determine whether goals and objectives have been achieved. Let's consider a hypothetical course entitled "Foundations of Clinical Practice."

One overall goal for Foundations of Clinical Practice is for the student to become a competent, compassionate, and ethical clinician. An objective related to that goal is for the student to develop basic skills in conducting and summarizing the patient interview. Strategies for helping students achieve this goal include lectures, small group discussion and practice, and interaction with simulated patients. Lectures address general communication skills, specific components of taking a history, and dealing with patients' emotions. Small group sessions provide students with multiple opportunities to practice these skills before they interact with simulated patients. Assessment strategies include evaluations by the simulated patients, written exam questions related to factual knowledge about elements of the history, and questions that require students to demonstrate that they know what questions to ask to characterize a symptom for a written case scenario.

Another example of an overall goal is to teach students to apply relevant basic and clinical science principles to the practice of medicine. One objective states that the course will help students integrate information learned in other courses in a clinically meaningful way. This is accomplished primarily through small group discussion in problem-based learning groups. Assessment includes facilitator evaluations, peer evaluations, written tests over the terminology, and a one-page essay question that asks students to write as though they were talking to the patient in the problem-based learning case in order to explain the diagnosis, explain what is causing the problem, describe how the lab tests and history confirmed the diagnosis, and tell the patient what to expect from the treatment.

The Learning Environment

How well students learn is influenced by a variety of factors. Their own prior knowledge and motivation are certainly important. Input from their fellow students, especially if instruction is designed to take advantage of collaborative learning, can also be important. The environment can also have a profound effect on learning. For example, is the physical environment arranged so that students have easy access to study space? Is the schedule organized to maximize student learning? Are services such as tutoring or study groups available for students who need them? Does the learning environment in the preclinical years minimize unnecessary competition? Do faculty members set realistic standards for what students are expected to achieve? During the clinical years, do faculty members and residents serve as role models in the compassionate and ethical treatment of patients? Do they demonstrate professionalism in interactions with colleagues? Creating a collaborative learning environment is particularly challenging in medical education, as students who are admitted to medical school often have gotten there because of individual achievement, not because they have been working in collaborative learning environments. Yet medicine is not practiced in isolation. Physicians must know how to work with other professionals and with their patients. So it is important to create a learning environment in which collaboration is encouraged.

Take Home Points

- Exponential growth in medical knowledge requires new approaches in medical education.
- Long-term retention of knowledge requires active processing of information and use of higher-order thinking skills.
- Students who have choices about their learning and can maintain intrinsic motivation will learn better and be able to apply their knowledge outside the classroom.
- Teachers have an important role in designing learning activities and assessment strategies that foster independent learning and higher-order thinking skills.
- Frequent feedback and reflection are important components in self-directed learning.
- Working in a supportive learning environment that reinforces self-directed learning and professional behavior can enhance student learning.

References

Commission on Behavioral and Social Sciences and Education, National Research Council (2000) How people learn. In: Brain, mind, experience, and school. National Academy Press, Washington, DC. Available via http://www.nap.edu

Kern DE, Thomas PA, Howard DM, Bass EB (1998) Curriculum development for medical education: a six-step approach. Johns Hopkins University Press, Baltimore

Marchese TJ (1998) The new conversations about learning insights from neuroscience and anthropology, cognitive science and workplace studies. In: New horizons for learning. Available via: http://www.newhorizons.org/lifelong/higher_ed/marchese.htm

Stiggins RJ, Rubel E, Quellmalz E (1988) Measuring thinking skills in the classroom, rev ed. National Education Assn Professional Library, West Haven

For Further Reading

Ferguson KJ (2005) Problem-based learning: let's not throw the baby out with the bathwater. Med Educ 39(4):352–353

This is an editorial responding to criticism of problem-based learning

Team Based Learning Collaborative, Website: http://www.tlcollaborative.org

This website is a great resource for those interested in learning more about team- based learning

Eva KW, Regehr G (2005) Self-assessment in the health professions: a reformulation and research agenda. Acad Med 80(10):S46–S54

This article reviews the evidence related to self-assessment, and recommends approaches for improving self-assessment

Chapter 2
Teaching Large Groups

William B. Jeffries

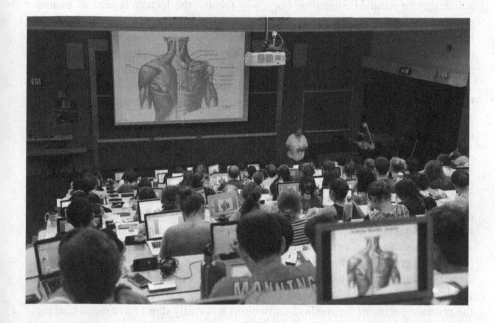

Abstract The 1 h lecture is a standard delivery mechanism for medical knowledge. In its traditional format, it has been shown to have serious limitations for domains of learning outside of knowledge transfer and students have difficulty maintaining attention throughout the delivery period. In this chapter, I examine some of the root causes of inattention and suggest ways to enhance learner engagement. In addition the

W.B. Jeffries, Ph.D. (✉)
Office of Medical Education, University of Vermont College of Medicine,
The Courtyard at Given, N117, 89 Beaumont Ave, Burlington, VT 05405, USA
e-mail: wbjeffri@uvm.edu

K.N. Huggett and W.B. Jeffries (eds.), *An Introduction to Medical Teaching*,
DOI 10.1007/978-94-017-9066-6_2, © Springer Science+Business Media Dordrecht 2014

steps for organizing and delivering a large group session are outlined and discussed. Important steps in an effective large group presentation include development of a lecture plan, use of a delivery style that enhances enthusiasm and optimization of pacing and content density. Other factors that increase lecture effectiveness include optimal audiovisual materials and the effective use of handouts. Finally, student learning and engagement can be enhanced through the incorporation of active learning methods within the session. Any lecture can be improved through the careful use of effective teaching methods and reflective use of student feedback.

Introduction

Despite many innovations in teaching and learning methods, the 1 h lecture remains a mainstay of medical education. For many faculty, the lecture is seen as an irreplaceable way to inform students about essential aspects of important subjects. However, for some the lecture format conjures up visions of students sitting long hours in their seats, passively listening to an expert expound on an esoteric topic. A large body of educational research has cast doubt on the amount of learning that actually takes place during a traditional lecture. The data show that while this format can be an effective way to transfer knowledge to students, it is not more effective than other methods (Bligh 2000). Further, the lecture is usually not the most optimal way to teach skills or change attitudes as compared to other methods. These findings are at the root of the movement to reduce the number of hours of lecture in the medical curriculum and replace them with the more "active" learning methods that are described in later chapters.

Despite these arguments, it has been reasoned that the lecture remains an effective and valuable format in medical education (Matheson 2008). There are several compelling reasons why lectures have not disappeared from the curricula of most medical schools. First, lectures offer a great economy of faculty time since other formats (e.g., small group teaching) require a larger number of faculty per activity. Second, since this format can be as good as any other for the simple transfer of information, it still makes sense to lecture. Third, many faculty automatically think of lectures as the primary engine of the medical curriculum and really don't have much training, experience or desire to teach in other ways. Finally, students also take this view of the curriculum and often expect to receive lectures as the primary vehicle for knowledge transfer and the exclusive source of material for knowledge assessments.

The goal of this chapter is to present ways of organizing and presenting a large group presentation that goes beyond the traditional boundaries of the lecture format. Our interest is in increasing student learning; this can be accomplished by modifying the format to increase engagement and introduce active learning methods. This will result in better learning, more engaged students and hopefully, better evaluations of your teaching. In this chapter, I will cover methods for constructing and delivering a 1 h presentation. Other large group methods that require formal outside preparation by the students, such as flipping the classroom and Team-Based Learning will be covered in subsequent chapters. I will assume you have been given the assignment of presenting a lecture for the first time in a large course. The examples will be specific to medical school, but the lessons will apply to any teaching you will be called upon to make in any large group setting.

Creating an Environment That Supports Learning

Before considering the construction of the optimal large group presentation, it is useful to think about how students learn in this environment. Schneider (1983) describe well established ideas of cognitive function that explain how students learn in the lecture hall. First, students must be attentive and determine what to pay attention to. Thus it is your job to make the lecture interesting and facilitate student focus. This includes attention to presentation style, varying the format and eliminating distracters. Next, students must organize this information into a pattern that is understandable to them. The lecturer must therefore pay particular attention to organization, context and prior knowledge of the students. In other words, the presentation must be designed to lead the students to the achievement of the objectives. Finally, students must take the information that is stored in their short-term memory and add it to their existing long-term knowledge base through a process known as **rehearsal**. This implies that the lecturer should enable rehearsal to occur by reinforcing important points, summing up and introducing learning exercises that ensure that new information is applied in context. It also means that you must avoid introducing elements that confound the learning process (e.g., changing topics too quickly, introducing too much or irrelevant information, etc.).

Developing a Large Group Presentation

Context

Before planning your large group presentation it is a good idea to consider the role of each presentation in the course. Since many medical school courses are team-taught, your presentation is likely to be interrelated to those of one or more instructors. Thus preparation should begin with a thoughtful discussion between the lecturer and course director. First, you should discuss the overall course objectives and assessment methods. Within that framework, what is your presentation supposed to accomplish? Second, you should determine the depth and scope of your area of responsibility. What do you expect the students to have learned (or to do) when the presentation is over? The answer to this question is best framed by writing out the objectives for the presentation (see below). Third, you should determine the relationship of the content assigned to you compared to that of the rest of the course. Is this topic related to other material in the course or curriculum? You should review the teaching materials presented by others on this topic to avoid gaps and

Table 2.1 Potential types of large group presentations and their purpose

Presentation of information about a subject. For example, a discussion of the etiology of heart failure
Development of critical thinking skills. For example, how to interpret epidemiological data about heart failure and apply that information to the diagnosis and treatment of a hypothetical patient
Demonstration of a procedure or clinical approach. For example, a demonstration of the use of the electrocardiogram in the diagnosis of heart ailments
Construction an academic argument. For example, influencing student attitudes regarding ethical policies of the distribution of donor hearts among transplant patients

Adapted from Newble and Cannon (2001)

redundancies of coverage. For example, if assigned a lecture on diabetes mellitus, you should consider how much carbohydrate metabolism should be included in your presentation. Fourth, you should become familiar with the instructional format of the course to ensure that your methods complement those used by others in the course. Within these boundaries, you should strive to include active learning methods to enhance student learning and maximize retention. In this vein, an appropriate question to ask is whether a lecture is the most appropriate format to use to cover the objectives. Other learning methods, found in later chapters in this book, may well prove to be the most optimal way to accomplish the course objectives. Assuming that this is not the case, planning for the lecture should continue as described below.

Purpose of the Presentation

Perhaps the most important question you can ask yourself when preparing a lecture for the first time is "what do I want my students to learn from this presentation?" Is it knowledge about a metabolic pathway? Is it how to perform a skill? It is how to critically interpret medical data? Is it to influence student attitudes about health policy? The answers to these question helps frame the objectives that you will construct to prepare the framework of the presentation. Further, they will influence how you present the material in the classroom. Table 2.1 shows some of the types of large group presentations that are classically used by medical teachers.

Development of the Content

If you are lecturing as part of a larger course, your broad goals and objectives are probably already defined. The content for your individual session is likely left up to you. It is therefore initially useful to consider the subject broadly and reflect on the topic and its many aspects without regard to the limitations imposed by the course. Depending on your own preferences, the ideas can be in the form of lists of topics, concept maps, outcome lists, taxonomies, etc. An approach I find helpful is create a list of the possible areas of instruction needed to cover a particular broad topic, and then organize them into a logical order. For example, let's say you have been assigned to teach the pharmacology of drugs used to treat heart failure:

Heart Failure Drugs

1. Normal cardiac function
2. Etiology of heart failure

    (a) Cellular
    (b) Organismal level

3. Strategies to combat heart failure
4. Drugs used to treat heart failure (repeat for each drug/class)

    (a) Chemistry
    (b) Pharmacokinetics
    (c) Pharmacodynamics

        (i)   Molecular and cellular effects
        (ii) Cardiac and hemodynamic effects
        (iii) Effects on other organs

    (d) Toxicity
    (e) Therapeutics

When organized in this way, you will quickly discover several things about your presentation:

1. Your outline overlaps other areas of the course/curriculum. Students may have already been exposed to normal cardiac function and etiology of heart failure. As stated earlier, a discussion with the other faculty in the course will help set your boundaries. However, your outline is still helpful since it helps define the prerequisite knowledge that students must have to understand your lecture. The stage is set for seamlessly integrating your presentation into the rest of the course.
2. There is too much to cover! If you did it correctly, you have created an exhaustive outline of the topic. Aside from areas outside the topic areas as discussed in #1, your outline helps you understand/define the scope of knowledge you expect to cover in the lecture. If this topic is your particular area of expertise, you will be tempted to include a plethora of the latest research findings, new hypotheses about cardiac failure, drugs on the horizon, etc. However, if your learners are first year medical students, your focus should be on covering the basics, saving the advanced material for another audience. One of the most common mistakes I see among new faculty is an overestimation of what students need to know in lecture. An advantage of developing a topic list is to help identify the essentials.
3. There is more than one way to organize the material. The organization of topics need not be too refined at this stage. Thus you should just make sure at this point that all your ideas are captured. Later, you will organize the material based on your objectives and the styles of the course.

4. The process has uncovered gaps in your own knowledge about the subject. One of the benefits of teaching is that it helps you develop your own knowledge of various subjects. Your knowledge gaps will prompt you to read more on the topic or consult a colleague to bring yourself up to date. You should also familiarize yourself with the relevant chapters from the assigned textbooks for the course. This will help you decide what information needs to be emphasized in class vs. that which is best left to the student to learn from the textbook.

At this stage you can then go back and compare your ideas with the specific objectives assigned for your course and lecture. Are the objectives appropriate? Are they achievable in the time allotted? Are they in the need of modification? You will likely conclude that the objectives need to be modified in some way. For example, if the objectives are not achievable in the time allotted, you will have to prioritize information to be presented (that which will be deferred for student reading or other out-of-class exercise, etc).

Development of the Lecture Plan

A well organized presentation improves learning and retention. What is the best way to organize a lecture? There is no best answer to this question; however, the organization should be dictated by several factors: the type of lecture (Table 2.1), the most logical sequence of information and the fostering of student attention, motivation and cognitive processing. Some common organizing principles are shown in Table 2.2.

Inductive approaches imply that a real world example is first presented and then the case specifics are used to generalize and develop the underlying theories. For example, a case could be presented in which a patient has developed some of the signs and symptoms of heart failure. This would allow a discussion of the mechanisms by which the patient developed this condition, and the principles of treatment. This would lead to a discussion of the specific drugs. **Deductive approaches** begin with a discussion of the underlying concepts (e.g., cellular physiology of the heart, hemodynamics, etc.) which lead to the discussion of specific cases. Time sequencing can be an effective approach (e.g., the development of heart failure treatment as a series of scientific breakthroughs) since the telling of stories promotes retention. Similarly, presenting a **pro vs. con** framework promotes retention because the academic argument presented promotes engagement and retention. A **familiar to unfamiliar** progression helps establish for the students the context into which the material fits.

Obviously, several of these principles may be used within the same lecture and all of them can convey information and enhance student learning. The plan will also be dictated by the type of large group session that is needed. If the purpose of the session is primarily the delivery of information or demonstration of a procedure, the objectives should be ordered in a simple outline format. If the purpose is the development of critical thinking skills or construction of an argument, then the organization and sequence has to be less defined to allow adjustments during the

Table 2.2 Ways to organize
a large group presentation

Inductive approaches
Problem to solution
Clinical case to diagnosis and treatment
Phenomenon to theory
Deductive approaches
Concept to application
General discussion to specific cases
Chaining of ideas (e.g., if A and B are true, then C must also be true)
Time sequence (e.g., chronological stories)
Pro vs. Con to solution
Familiar to unfamiliar (what students know to what they don't know)

Adapted from McKeachie and Svinicki (2006, p. 63)

teaching process. In this latter case the number of objectives also must be scaled back since the development of skills and attitudes needs time for development during the class period. Most importantly, regardless of the plan used, the students must be made aware of the organizational structure of the lecture to avoid confusion and enhance their ability to process information.

Presenting a Large Group Session

Using one or more of the formats outlined in the previous section, you should present a session that is designed to promote a learning-enabled environment. This means you will enhance attention, and use strategies to enhance cognitive function.

Planning the Beginning and the End

A great way to increase attention and instill student confidence is to have a well planned beginning to your lecture. In your first lecture, it is a good idea to introduce yourself and briefly discuss your larger role in the school (e.g., "I am a neuroscientist who researches the coordination of skeletal muscle movement by the brain, which is why I was chosen to discuss Parkinson's disease"). A brief, general outline of what will be covered is often the next step. It will aid learning if the student's understand the framework of your talk in advance. It is convenient to use the learning objectives in the outline to clarify their importance. Depending on the type of lecture, the next step may be to address the gap between the student's current knowledge and that needed to understand the subject (e.g., "You all have an excellent understanding of carbohydrate metabolism. Today we will attempt to apply that knowledge to the understanding of the etiology of Diabetes Mellitus"). Alternatively, you may use this opportunity to introduce a case or open-ended problem, which will then form the basis for the content to come. The ending of the lecture should also be well planned. Here is it often best to summarize the most salient points of the lecture. This will aid in student rehearsal and provide them with a focus for later review. Time for final questions should also be allotted. This should include time for students to approach you immediately after the lecture in case they are uncomfortable asking their question in front of the class.

Projecting Enthusiasm

Students respond to the enthusiasm of the instructor with increased attentiveness (Bligh 2000). There are many ways to project enthusiasm. The easiest is to move around the room and directly engage the audience. Conversely, the quickest way to induce classroom boredom is to use a monotone presentation and stand directly behind the podium. This is particularly true in a large lecture hall where students may not easily see your facial expressions. In this case it is important to get out from behind the podium and mingle with the audience. Make eye contact with specific students and vary your vocal expression. A technique that I use is to arrive early and scan the class photo (usually available from the course director or Office of Medical Education) to identify several students in the audience. During the lecture, you can call them by name and engage them specifically. Be careful to do this in a non-threatening manner! The judicious use of humor can also help maintain attention. If you are not comfortable with verbal witticisms, you can show a humorous cartoon. Relevant anecdotes also can enhance arousal and improve retention. Such overtures let the students see you are engaged and interested in a rapport with them. Student attention and engagement are bound to dramatically rise.

A note of caution is needed when discussing enthusiasm. Although enthusiasm does promote learning in the classroom, studies have shown that excellent engagement alone can be perceived as excellent learning by the students, irrespective of the actual value of the content (Ware and Williams 1975; Murray 1997). In these studies, a fictional "Dr. Fox" gave lectures with either a high degree of enthusiasm (movement, vocal emphasis, humor, etc.) or low enthusiasm (unexpressive, monotone delivery) and varying degrees of meaningful content. As expected, it was found that student learning was greatest in high enthusiasm/high content lectures. However, student ratings revealed that they considered a high enthusiasm teacher to be effective regardless of the level of content. Ware and Williams (1975) called this the "Dr. Fox Effect." Thus, students appreciate the entertainment value of the lecture and the instructor may come to an erroneous conclusion as to his/her effectiveness based on student feedback. One should always keep in mind that while enthusiasm is an effective tool to promote attention, challenging and meaningful content must also be introduced to produce student learning (Table 2.3).

Table 2.3 Tips for engagement	Arrive early; stay late
	Move around room, delivering various points from different locations
	Make eye contact with students
	Call students by name
	Make expressive gestures and body movements
	Vary the tone of your voice
	Ask questions
	Use humor
	Vary presentation style

Pacing and Density of Content

The speed at which material is introduced is a critical factor that influences learning. Often students are unfamiliar with material being introduced and must build their knowledge base over the course of the lecture. Studies of lecture pacing revealed that students hardly ever complain if the lecturer has a delivery that is too slow (Bligh 2000, p. 223). On the other hand, if a lecture is paced too quickly, the ability of students to build concepts is overwhelmed and learning is impaired dramatically. The pace of delivery is directly related to the amount of information to be covered. In health science education it is common to see an instructor attempt to cover 80 or 90 detailed slides in a 50 min presentation. In this case, you can expect very little long term learning to occur. The speed necessary to deliver material of this density will reduce attention, depress cognition, inhibit effective note taking and decrease learning. Thus you must limit the amount of material in your presentation and focus it on major points to be remembered. If you have been assigned too much material and too little time it will be necessary to employ additional learning methods, such as assigned reading or homework problems to accomplish the learning objectives. The important thing to remember (and stress with the course director) is that simply speeding up the presentation is not a viable option.

Attention Span vs. Lecture Length

Some authors suggest that despite an enthusiastic presentation, student attention in the lecture hall can wane dramatically after only 10–15 min (summarized in Bligh 2000 and McKeachie and Svinicki 2006). While other authors suggest that this decline in attention span varies widely (Wilson and Korn 2007), even highly motivated learners can begin to squirm in their seats and become distracted well before the lecture is over. Lecture length has another negative impact on learning: **interference**. Since there is a finite capacity to short-term memory, new material just learned can displace material learned just minutes earlier. This combination of reduced attention and interference can potentially create a gap in learning, particularly in the middle of the lecture. Fortunately there are measures you can take to prevent this. It has been shown that varying the format can restore attention. Further, providing opportunities for rehearsal of short-term memories into long-term learning can effectively combat interference. Therefore no more than 10–15 min should pass before summing up (which aids rehearsal) and introducing an active learning exercise to promote "hard coding" of student learning experiences. Some suggested exercises are included in the next section.

Getting Feedback

Even the best lecturers can lose their audience. I have witnessed well thought-out, enthusiastic lectures that were unfortunately delivered at a level well beyond the student's learning capacity. Thus it is imperative to obtain feedback from your learners during the presentation to determine that they are actually following and comprehending your presentation. The easiest way to get this information is to ask at the end of each major point if there are any questions.

This often elicits no response, especially in the large lecture hall. This may be because everyone understands, but it may be that some students are too intimidated in the presence of their peers to admit that they don't understand something. One of the ways to approach this challenge is to create buzz groups (see next section) which can be used to identify the "muddiest point". Another newer solution is via the use of an audience response system. This system, described in Chap. 10, can elicit anonymous answers to questions posed by you during lecture. This approach serves a dual purpose. First, you can obtain real-time feedback as to whether students comprehend your lecture. Second, you are allowing rehearsal of the most important concepts during lecture, which enhances the likelihood of retention.

Handouts

Studies have shown that note-taking increases learning and retention of the material presented in large group formats. Thus it is a good idea to prepare handouts that lend themselves to note taking and reinforcement of the lessons given in class. A familiar format is a general outline that can be filled in with specifics during the lecture. Another common format is to provide an exact copy of your presentation slides in paper or electronic form to the students. This allows students to annotate your presentation in the lecture hall. Both of these formats are easily posted into online content management systems and allow students to use their computers to take detailed, typed notes on your presentation. One should beware three things when preparing handouts for use in class. First, make sure that you have not provided too much information, such as long, detailed bullet points. This discourages note taking and encourages the instructor to read them off in the lecture, reducing engagement. Second, make sure that slides that are easily seen when projected are also easily read when printed. Slides featuring detailed histology can become amorphous

Table 2.4 Effective slide presentations

Avoid dark background with white letters. This requires lower room lighting, which encourages dozing

Don't put too much information on a single slide. The number of bullet points should not exceed 4–5. The font size should be as large as possible, at least 18 pt

Ensure that figures are legible when projected

Do not put conflicting information formats on a single slide (e.g., a graph with bullet point explanation)

Bullet points should not be detailed sentences. Rather, they should be heading names that allow for expansion in class

Allow 2–3 min per slide

Allow for other educational elements to be included in the presentation. A single lecture of 50 PowerPoint slides is a sure way to lose the student's attention

smudges, graph legends can disappear and complex biochemical reactions can be undecipherable when rendered as six black and white images per page. Thus, it is worth taking the time to look over how the handout of your presentation will look before entering the lecture hall. Finally, ensure that you have secured copyright permissions for figures and materials you will include in your handouts. Once in the student's hands, these documents fall into the public domain and you are responsible for the content in them.

Audiovisual Materials

Audiovisual materials introduced in a large group presentation should complement the presentation and promote active learning. The most common presentation method in large group settings is the "slide show," in which the instructor can project text and images to illustrate the important points of the lecture. The physical slide has given way to electronic presentation formats, most commonly Microsoft PowerPoint. Some tips for an effective slide show can be found in Table 2.4. More specific guidelines for use of PowerPoint© can be found in Chap. 10.

Other audiovisual materials can include videos, demonstrations, white or black board, models, etc. The key to the use of these materials is that they are relevant, visible at a distance, and easily comprehended in the lecture hall. With regard to this latter point, I recall a colleague who developed a detailed animation of a physiological process for presentation in class, but the students who viewed it could not comprehend it's complexity in the allotted time. Audiovisual materials should help explain things, not provide barriers to understanding.

Active Learning Methods in the Lecture Hall

As stated previously, a key to increasing learning in the large group setting is involving the students with active, rather than passive methods. When introducing active learning methods into the lecture hall, you may meet some resistance. Some students do not understand the need for active learning methods. A question you may sometimes get is "why can't you just tell us what we need to remember for the exam?" In this case you should state that the purpose of the presentation is to learn about the material IN THE CLASSROOM. Tell them that valid educational data show that sitting for an hour just listening is not the best way to learn. Thus other elements of active learning MUST be incorporated into the hour. Finally, you must ensure that your assessment questions on examinations require more than just rote memorization. If students are made aware of this, there will be great interest in active learning in the classroom. Students who initially disapproved of these techniques have regaled me years later with stories about how they still remember lecture points solidified by active learning methods. In this Section I will introduce some ideas for incorporating active learning into a large group session. The list is not exhaustive, but is intended to start you in a search for the best methods to complement your own presentation style.

Lecture Respites

The simplest way to promote student learning during a lecture is to provide a short respite from lecture. This can be done every 10–15 min to maintain student arousal. One way is to say "at this point I will stop for a **note check** I want you to review your notes and then ask me questions if needed." This simple device allows students to begin to make sense of the lecture, clarify points they don't understand, and process the information into long-term memory. You can help the process along by suggesting areas to focus on in their brief review, or present or ask a question yourself for them to go and answer from their notes. The solitary review should last only about a minute, to discourage social chatting with neighbors.

Small Group Activities

The best way to overcome the limitations of a large group is to break up the class into smaller units that can engage in other activities. **Buzz groups** are a form of peer learning that can be introduced into any large group presentation. The instructor poses a problem, and then divides the class in groups of about four students each to quickly solve it. In my lectures I simply ask the students to turn to their neighbors and discuss the problem. After a short interval (2–3 min) the instructor calls on a reporter from selected groups to present their answer. The question can be subdivided so that different groups have different parts of the question, which can promote a class-wide discussion to synthesize the best solution. Further questions can be introduced during the discussion by the instructor to promote further discussion. I sometimes create impromptu buzz groups if I feel that the class is having difficulty understanding a concept. The buzz group format is quite adaptable and can occupy just a few minutes or an extended time as needed. A variant of the buzz group is the **"Think-Pair-Share"** or **"Pair Discussion."** Here students work on a problem or discussion question of limited complexity by themselves for 1–5 min (**think**), then form a working pair with their nearest neighbor (**pair**). The discussion time allotted is also short (about 3–5 min), and the instructor calls on a limited number of pairs to report and discuss their answer (**share**). Despite the limited discussion period, all students work on the problem with a peer and derive benefits from actively applying their new knowledge in this format. The pair discussion format can also be combined with the note check strategy described above in which students determine if they have missed anything, discuss the salient points and ensure that they both agree on what was important.

Reading or problem solving activities can also be attempted in a large group setting. There are many variations to this format, but it usually the assignment of a specific reading, viewing a video vignette or problem-solving task. Students complete the tasks individually for a defined period of time, then break into pairs or small groups for discussion and resolution of problems. Then the groups report to the large group during a general large group discussion facilitated by the instructor. There are many possible variants to this scenario.

Classroom Survey Techniques

Classroom survey techniques are methods to poll the class about their preferences on certain topics or answers to questions during the session. This can be done by eliciting a simple show of hands, by holding up numbered cards or by use of sophisticated audience response systems as described in Chap. 10. This format can create a lively and interactive environment to promote learning in a large group. The most common approach to the method is to periodically ask the students a multiple choice question and to quickly tally the answers from the class. There are tangible benefits to both the instructor and the student. The instructor receives instant feedback as to the comprehension of the class and can adjust the content and pace of the lecture accordingly. Disparate answers can also be used to generate a class discussion. For the student, attentiveness is improved and knowledge gained during the lecture is directly applied to promote long-term retention. Use of an automated audience response system can greatly facilitate this process. In addition to instant feedback, the audience response system offers the advantage of anonymous responses, integration with presentation software, individual tracking and grading of responses and immediate graphical display of the results. When using any classroom survey technique, the instructor must be prepared to alter the course of the presentation based on the level of comprehension of the students. A final use of classroom survey techniques worth discussing is for assessment. Short quizzes can be introduced at the end of lectures to reinforce learning. Conversely, quizzes can be introduced at the beginning of each lecture to assess prior knowledge or to ensure completion of the reading assignment.

Reflective Techniques

A number of techniques exist (see Angelo and Cross 1993) that call on the student to directly apply new knowledge in the class to increase comprehension and allow higher level of learning. For example, the two (or one) minute paper or "half sheet response" is an effective way for students to synthesize the knowledge gained during the large group session (McKeachie and Svinicki 2006, p. 256). Typically, the students are asked to take 2 min at the end of class to produce a short essay explaining the most salient point(s) of the lecture. Other topics that could be tasked include "Give an example of this concept' or "discuss treatment options for this disease," etc. This aids in retention and understanding of the material. The essay can be for self evaluation or the instructor can collect them for grading. A variant is where the instructor stops the class and asks them to produce a 1 or 2 min essay on an assigned topic that relates to the lecture material. A related technique is the One-Sentence Summary, where the instructor asks each student to prepare a declarative sentence that summarizes a key point. Directed Paraphrasing is another variant in which students are asked to paraphrase a specific part of a lesson in their own words. This can be done in written form or verbally after allowing a short reflective period. One final example is the student generated test question, in which students are asked to develop a "one best answer" question about a specific point in the presentation. These questions can be used in several ways: they can be graded by the instructor, answered by neighboring students, compiled into a quiz given prior to the next teaching session, posted on the class bulletin board, etc. Several other examples of effective techniques are detailed by Angelo and Cross (1993). In each case, the techniques serve to increase engagement and reinforce student learning in the classroom.

Games

Some faculty are able to introduce active learning in students by catering to their competitive nature. In the game format, quiz questions are introduced and student teams compete to answer them. Scores may be kept and nominal prizes may even be awarded to the best teams. There are many variations to this format. Small competitions can be held during the last 5 min of the session, or entire sessions can be given over to review a course section via this approach. The biggest advantage of the game approach is that it creates a fun, energy filled environment for learning. The primary disadvantages are the time it takes to conduct the sessions and the loss of focus that can occur in the game environment.

Getting Beyond Boundaries of Lecturing

At the beginning of this chapter I stated that although lectures are an educational mainstay, active learning is much more feasible in other educational formats. Recognizing this, educators are beginning to modify the large group setting to

Table 2.5 Common mistakes to avoid in large group teaching

Lack of engagement: monotone presentation from behind the podium
Information overload: too many slides, too fast paced, too many objectives
Poorly thought out beginning and ending
Simply reading bullet points off of the slides
Inadequate knowledge of context of your presentation: gaps, redundancies and conflicting information
No time for assimilation and reflection
Not knowing your learners: teaching is too elementary or beyond their comprehension
Entertaining, but not informative: beware the Dr. Fox effect!

reduce or eliminate lectures and maximize the opportunity for active learning and peer teaching. Two related formats warrant introduction and are the subjects of chapters in this book: flipping the classroom and Team-Based Learning. In both cases, students are responsible for completing assignments before coming to class to ensure a baseline knowledge acquisition. In the large group, students complete assignments or assessments that apply the knowledge, leading to higher levels of learning and better retention. A full discussion of the flipped classroom can be found in Chap. 4 and TBL is introduced in Chap. 6.

A Final Word

Developing and delivering an effective lecture can be a daunting challenge. It is important to review the feedback gained from students and peers and to continue to improve the quality and the amount of learning that takes place in your sessions. Table 2.5 summarizes some of the common pitfalls that can befall even the most experienced lecturers. Further information on diagnosing lecture problems can be found in a humorous but informative paper by McLaughlin and Mandin (2001). Chapter 16 discusses in detail how evaluation data to improve your teaching.

Hopefully this chapter has provided both a framework for engaging students actively in the large group setting and a way of avoiding common mistakes. Additional resources are provided below to provide an in-depth treatment of this topic.

References

Angelo TA, Cross KP (1993) Classroom assessment techniques: a handbook for college teachers. Jossey-Bass, San Francisco

Bligh DA (2000) What's the use of lectures? Jossey-Bass, New York

Matheson C (2008) The educational value and effectiveness of lectures. Clin Teach 5:219–221

McKeachie WJ, Svinicki M (2006) McKeachie's teaching tips. Strategies, research, and theory for college and university teachers. Houghton Mifflin, Boston

McLaughlin K, Mandin H (2001) A schematic approach to diagnosing and resolving lecturalgia. Med Educ 35:1135–1142

Murray HG (1997) Effective teaching behavior in the college classroom. In: Perry RP, Smart JC (eds) Effective teaching in higher education: research and practice. Agathon Press, New York, pp 171–204

Newble D, Cannon R (2001) A handbook for medical teachers, 4th edn. Kluwer Academic Publishers, Dordrecht

Schneider FB (1983) A practical handbook for college teachers. Little, Brown and Company, Boston

Ware JE, Williams RG (1975) The Dr. Fox effect: a study of lecturer effectiveness and ratings of instruction. J Med Educ 50:149–156

Wilson K, Korn JH (2007) Attention during lectures: beyond ten minutes. Teach Psychol 34(2):85–89

Chapter 3
Teaching in Small Groups

Kathryn N. Huggett

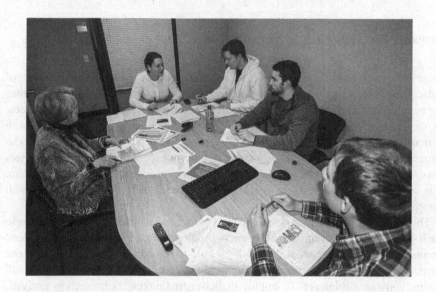

Abstract There are many unique benefits to teaching and learning in small groups. Recognizing this, many medical schools have increased the amount of time devoted to small group learning. Very few faculty members, however, have received formal instruction for leading small groups. To ensure effective small group teaching, you must first understand the purpose for the small group and then select activities for the group that will enable learners to achieve the learning objectives. Understanding both your role as the teacher and the dynamics of the group will help you foster participation among group members. This chapter offers practical suggestions for preparing for and facilitating small groups.

K.N. Huggett, Ph.D. (✉)
Office of Medical Education, Creighton University School of Medicine,
2500 California Plaza, Criss III, Room 463, Omaha, NE 68178, USA
e-mail: kathrynhuggett@creighton.edu

K.N. Huggett and W.B. Jeffries (eds.), *An Introduction to Medical Teaching*,
DOI 10.1007/978-94-017-9066-6_3, © Springer Science+Business Media Dordrecht 2014

Introduction

There are many unique benefits to teaching and learning in small groups. Recognizing this, many medical schools have increased the amount of time devoted to small group learning. Very few faculty members, however, have received formal instruction for facilitating small groups. This has contributed to misperceptions about the value of small group learning. It also explains why many faculty members do not feel confident teaching in this setting. Teaching in small groups can be satisfying and even inspiring, but it can also be time consuming and dispiriting when difficulties arise. To ensure effective small group teaching, you must first understand the purpose for the small group and then select activities for the group that will enable learners to achieve the learning objectives. Understanding both your role as the teacher and the dynamics of the group will help you foster participation among group members.

Reasons for Teaching in Small Groups

There are many advantages to teaching in small groups. The smaller number of participants means that you will have an opportunity to know your students' names and become familiar with their knowledge, interests, and prior learning experiences. As the course progresses, you will be able to conduct ongoing assessment, both formal and informal, of learners' comprehension and application of the course content. This will enhance your efforts to target your teaching strategies. Learners in a small group benefit because they have increased contact time with their instructor. You will find learners are often more comfortable asking questions during small group sessions than larger lectures.

There are significant educational outcomes associated with teaching and learning in small groups. The small number of learners promotes engagement between learners, the instructor, and the content. You will be able to introduce activities that require learners to move beyond the recall and recognition of concepts. When teaching in small groups, you can ask learners to employ higher-order thinking skills such as analysis, reasoning, and criticism. To do this, you might create opportunities for learners to demonstrate problem-solving skills. These activities will allow you to assess if your learners are able to apply new knowledge and concepts. Similarly, the small group provides a venue for learners to rehearse material they have read or learned in lectures. Westberg and Jason (1996, p. 7) have referred to this as learners' opportunity to "build and 'metabolize' knowledge." In the small group, learners can pose questions about the material, discuss inconsistencies, and propose applications of the material. This will help learners to see and understand the connections between the material in your course and others in their area of study. As the small group facilitator, you can provide learners with information about the context for the material and its relevance. This will also assist learners in understanding and applying new knowledge.

Small groups offer two additional educational outcomes. First, the small size and increased engagement of the group promote reflection on learning. Recognizing what you have learned, what you do not know, and what you still need to know is essential to becoming a professional. This is the foundation of lifelong learning, and you can model this for your learners. In addition to fostering reflection on learning, small groups provide learners with opportunities to develop the interpersonal skills necessary to work in a group or team setting. This is becoming more important as health care is increasingly provided by teams of diverse professionals. Participation in small groups can improve skills in active listening, presentation, negotiation, group leadership, and cooperative problem solving.

Definition of Small Group Teaching

Teaching and learning can occur anywhere, but some learning objectives are best achieved by small group teaching. Small groups are often used to complement lecture-based courses. When this occurs, the small group meets to discuss the lectures or readings. Small groups are also ideal for working through cases that integrate material from the lectures or other required courses. Small group teaching and learning also occur in problem-based curricula and laboratory courses. Each of these small group activities presents unique considerations for planning and teaching, and will be discussed elsewhere in this book.

The size of small groups can vary considerably in medical education. Research has demonstrated that groups composed of five to eight learners are the optimal size for Problem-Based Learning (PBL) groups (Westberg and Jason 1996). This range has been cited as favorable for other small group experiences as well (Jacques 2003). However, limitations posed by physical space and faculty availability lead many medical schools to organize small groups with more than eight learners. The size of the group is not the only determinant of small group teaching. In medical education it is not unusual to find learners in a small group session listening to a lecture given by the instructor. This is not small group teaching. Newble and Cannon (2001) cite three important characteristics of small group teaching:

- Active participation.
- Purposeful activity.
- Face-to-face contact.

Active Participation

To realize the educational benefits of small group teaching, it is essential that all members of the group participate. The small group size will ensure there is time and opportunity for all learners to contribute to the discussion or activity. This is important because you will want to assess each learner's development in knowledge and understanding. Greater participation among all group members also ensures sufficient opportunities for learners to hone their communication and team skills. If the group is larger than eight learners, you can still use small group teaching methods, but will need to be both creative and intentional in planning the activities. Some of the techniques for teaching in small groups can be accomplished successfully if you create multiple subgroups within the existing small group (Jacques 2003). The effort will be worthwhile, however, and students have identified active student participation and group interaction as a characteristic of an effective small group (Steinert 2004).

Purposeful Activity

We have all had the unpleasant experience of participating in a meeting or small group session where there is no agenda or plan for the activity. The lack of purpose is frustrating, and contributes to the feeling that our time was misspent. This is not unlike the experience learners have when small group teaching is not organized around purposeful activity. Not surprising, medical students have identified clinical relevance and integration, and adherence to small group goals as essential to effective small groups (Steinert 2004). The purpose, or goal, you create for each session may be broad, but then the session and discussion should be organized to accomplish this goal. In addition to determining the content focus of the session, you will also want to think about the other learning outcomes that can be achieved during the session, such as critical appraisal of the literature or team negotiation. Too much activity can also become a problem, especially if it limits participation by all group members. Developing a plan for each session will help ensure that learners remain engaged and that the goals of the session are met. A small group session plan is also helpful for small group leaders who are less experienced or less skilled in small group teaching. The plan will provide guidance on how to structure the session activities and manage time effectively.

Face-to-Face Contact

While recent advances in instructional technology have fostered effective strategies for online or e-learning, the type of small group teaching described in this chapter requires face-to-face contact. A synchronous, or "real-time," discussion requires that learners demonstrate presentation and other communication skills while working collaboratively to apply knowledge and solve a new problem. As the instructor, you will be able to observe these skills and also learners' non-verbal communication skills such as eye contact and posture. Likewise, learners need to be able to see the other members of their group, and it may be necessary to reconfigure the room so this can occur. If possible, reserve seminar-style rooms or rooms with furniture that can be re-arranged easily.

Preparing for the Small Group Session

Preparing for small group teaching begins like preparing for any other type of teaching. First, determine the learning objectives for the session. One way to do this is to write a list of outcomes, where each statement begins "By the end of this session, learners will be able to..." As you fill in the blank with a knowledge, skill or attitude objective, remember that the small group session is an appropriate place to ask learners to demonstrate higher-order thinking skills such as reasoning and critical appraisal. Taxonomies, such as those developed by Bloom (1956) and revised by Anderson et al. (2001), provide guidance on classifying learning objectives. Consult Chap. 1 of this book for a review of learning objectives and taxonomies of thinking skills, including an overview of a taxonomy developed by Quellmaz (Stiggins et al. 1988). Review your list of objectives periodically, and ask yourself if the small group is the best place to teach and learn each objective.

After you have determined the learning objectives for the session, review the characteristics of the learners enrolled in the small group. Is this course their first introduction to the subject matter? Can you assume they have all completed similar core courses or prerequisites? The answers to these questions will help you determine expectations for their participation. Are you acquainted with the learners already? Are they acquainted with each other? This is important to know before asking learners to work collaboratively or discuss sensitive topics.

The next step in planning the small group session is to determine the structure for the session. First, review the amount of time allotted for the session and the total number of sessions for the topic and course. Then establish which objectives will be addressed in each session. If you are responsible for planning a session within a series of small group sessions, review your colleagues' plans to ensure your coverage of the content is complementary and not redundant. Next, determine the appropriate activity for teaching and learning the objectives. For example, you might begin the session by inviting learners to discuss points that were unclear in the recent lecture. Another option is to open the session with an interesting finding or news item that relates to the course. Then the session might continue with discussion of a case and conclude with time for learners to reflect on the case and ask questions. To ensure that you accomplish all planned activities within the allotted amount of time, develop an agenda for each session. An example of an agenda for a small group discussion session in a medical ethics course is illustrated in Table 3.1.

Do not feel that the agenda or schedule cannot be changed, however. You will need to adapt the plan as the session unfolds. Some tasks may require less time than you estimated and it will be appropriate to begin the next activity earlier than planned. During some sessions, you may need to re-allocate time to clarify difficult concepts or address questions that arise. The outline should be a guide and not a rigid schedule. Over time, you will feel more comfortable adapting the schedule.

Table 3.1 Agenda for a small group session in a medical ethics course

Activity	Time (min)
Attendance and announcements	5
Student presentation of ethics case	10
Presenters identify two unresolved ethical questions	5
Group discussion of the case and questions	20
Student presentation of case and commentaries from textbook	10
Group discussion of the case and commentaries	20
Wrap-up and review of deadlines for upcoming assignments	5
Total session time	75

Leading the Small Group Session

Thoughtful preparation before teaching small groups will lead to well-organized sessions that are integrated into the curriculum for the course. However, careful planning can only ensure part of the success of teaching in small groups. As a small group facilitator, you will soon find that your leadership and the dynamics of the group are critical elements.

Attributes of an Effective Small Group Teacher

Effective small group teachers are well prepared for each session and are acquainted with goals and objectives for the entire course. Take time to become familiar with the lecture topics in the course, especially those that relate to the cases or topics discussed in the small group session. The time you spend preparing in advance of each small group will improve the organization and flow of each session. You may also find you spend less time on learners' questions about the administrative details of the course and more time on learning. How you conduct yourself during the session may be even more important than how much you prepare. Your primary focus is the learner, and not the content or activity. Effective small group teachers demonstrate interest in and respect for their learners. One way to do this is to introduce yourself at the first session, and briefly tell learners about your role in the course or other responsibilities in medical education. Also, remember to let learners know how to reach you if they have questions outside of the small group session. Another way to demonstrate respect for your learners is to recognize that each small group will be composed of learners with different backgrounds, personalities, and learning styles. These shape learners' responses to the tasks and roles that are assigned within the group. Two sources for information about personality types are the Myers-Briggs Type Indicator (1995) and Keirsey Temperament Sorter (1998). Both instruments provide insight into an individual's predispositions and attitudes. These tests do not assess ability or psychological traits; instead, results from these profiles can help to explain how individuals differ when making decisions or obtaining new information. To better understand differences in individuals' preferences for learning, consult David Kolb's Learning Styles Inventory (LSI) (1984). The LSI is a well-known model of learning styles based upon a cycle of learning that describes how all people learn.

While effective small group teachers appreciate the differences among learners, they also understand that their own teaching and learning preferences may differ from those of their students. Our preferences even influence our leadership style in the small group setting. For example, some teachers are highly-skilled at lecturing to large groups. They may prefer to teach and learn in this type of environment where attention is focused on the individual instructor and there is minimal inter-action with the group. For this individual, moving to the interactive, small-group setting can be challenging. It is not unusual for this type of teacher to revert to lecturing within the small group, especially if they perceive group activity as difficult to manage. Acknowledging these preferences for teaching and learning will help you to recognize when your own style begins to overshadow the learner-centered approach. When Steinert (2004) queried medical students about the advice they would give to small group tutors, their recommendations included "remember that we are only students, be excited to be there, and please don't lecture in the small group."

Effective small group teachers also promote a learner-centered approach to small group teaching by providing frequent, formative feedback. This type of feedback helps learners to assess their progress and make changes while the course is still in progress. Feedback should be specific so that learners recognize which element of their performance should be improved or, in the case of positive feedback, continued. Specific examples and constructive suggestions for improvement will enhance the quality of feedback.

Conditions for an Effective Small Group Session

Successful small group sessions rarely occur simply because of an enthusiastic teacher or motivated learners. Effective, learner-centered groups require multiple conditions for success. First, each group should agree upon ground rules such as no late arrivals, texting, or criticism during idea-generating activities. If students are new to small group learning, you may want to explain that all learners have a right to participate, but they can pass or occasionally request assistance from a classmate. Likewise, you may want to discuss rules to limit speaking too frequently during the sessions. These basic rules will help to promote respect among group members and develop group cohesion. If you engage learners in determining expectations for peer behavior, you will find they are more invested in the group and more likely to adhere to the group's norms for behavior. Second, each small group should discuss clear guidelines for participation and assessment. As the small group teacher, you should explain your expectations for participation and how this contributes to the evaluation of learners' performance. When learners are confused about the criteria for assessment, they may become anxious and less willing to participate. Take time to clarify the roles that learners will play in the small group, such as presenter or reporter, and explain how often learners will change roles. Likewise, explain to learners which resources they are responsible for bringing to the session so that they arrive prepared. Small group sessions are less likely to become unfocused or unproductive when learners are prepared and informed about the purpose and expectations for the session.

Finally, small groups generally flourish in an environment that is cooperative and collaborative, rather than competitive. While occasional friendly competition, such as a quiz-show activity, might engage the group and promote collegiality, a pervasive environment of cut-throat competition will stifle participation. As a small group teacher, you can develop activities that require collaboration and should intervene when an overly competitive learner seeks control of the session or resources. More challenging is managing students' reluctance to participate if they fear revealing knowledge deficits in front of their peers. This is often the case early in their education when they have not yet spent a lot of time with their classmates. As an instructor you can assist by developing activities that encourage pairs or trios to work together before contributing to the larger group discussion.

Understanding Group Dynamics

Small groups in medical education share many characteristics with small groups or teams organized for other professional purposes. Scholtes et al. (2000), building upon earlier work by Bruce Tuckman (1965), describe a four-stage process that all groups undergo. This model is useful for anticipating learners' attitudes and behaviors in your small group. In the first stage, called **forming**, group members feel excitement, anticipation and optimism. Some learners may also experience anxiety or suspicion about the work ahead. Remember that students, especially in the first year of medical school, are accustomed to being successful in academic settings. They may be hesitant to appear unprepared or unskilled in front of peers with whom they have not yet established friendships and trust. Scholtes encourages leaders to help the group members become acquainted and develop rules during the forming stage. In the second stage, **storming**, learners may exhibit resistance to tasks or express concern about excessive work. Arguments between group members may arise. The effective small group teacher will help learners resolve these issues. In the third stage, **norming**, groups demonstrate acceptance of small group members. A developing sense of cohesion fosters discussion and constructive criticism. During this stage, effective small group teachers will promote collaboration. The final stage, **performing**, is characterized by the group's ability to work through problems. Sholtes notes that group members now have a better understanding of others' strengths and weaknesses. The effective small group teacher will monitor progress and provide feedback during this stage. Groups will differ in how much time they spend in each stage of the process, but will ideally spend most of their time in the latter stages. As the small group teacher, you can observe the group and facilitate appropriate transitions between stages.

Small Group Discussion Methods

There are many approaches to teaching in small groups but the most successful ones are organized around a purposeful activity. Two highly-structured approaches, Problem-Based Learning (PBL) and Team-Based Learning (TBL), are discussed in Chaps. 5 and 6, respectively. In medical education, the structured case discussion is a common approach. Learners present a patient case and then work together to accomplish tasks such as developing a diagnosis and management plan. As described earlier in Table 3.1, a structured case discussion session typically allows the majority of time for individual learner presentations and group discussion. A limited amount of time is allocated for the small group leader to open and conclude the session and, as needed, clarify aspects of the case that are unclear. The structured approach to the case discussion means that time is allocated for each task. This ensures that the discussion is organized and stays on course.

While the case is a common stimulus for small group discussion in the health sciences, there are other materials that can be used to organize or initiate discussion. Examples of stimulus material include:

- A brief audio or video presentation.
- Visual material pertinent to the discussion (e.g., diagnostic images or charts).
- Material available via the Internet.
- A journal article or other thought-provoking written material.
- A real or standardized patient.
- Observation of a role play.
- A "one minute paper" that learners write and then share.
- A brief multiple choice test.

Variations in Small Group Teaching

In addition to case discussion, there are other methods that can be used in teaching small groups. When you prepare to teach in a small group setting, consider the purpose or goal for the session, and then select a technique that is best suited to achieving the learning objectives. Sometimes it is useful to introduce a different technique to promote learner interest and engagement. Other times it may be useful to use a different technique to overcome a challenging group dynamic.

1. *Paired (one-to-one) discussion:* The paired, or one-to-one discussion is easy to facilitate and effective for many topics. To use this technique, organize the group

into pairs. As the small group teacher, you can participate in this activity as well. One member of each pair should talk on the assigned topic for 3–5 min, without interruption. The roles are then reversed and the other member of the pair becomes the discussant. You may need to remind the group periodically that questions and comments should be held until later in the session. After the pairs have concluded their one-to-one discussion, the group reconvenes and each person provides a brief summary of the comments made by their partner. This technique helps learners to develop listening, summarization, and presentation skills. The paired discussion is effective as an introductory ice breaker, where learners use the discussion and presentation time to meet and learn more about their colleagues. This small group technique is also valuable for discussing topics that are emotionally-charged or controversial. By assigning learners to pairs and enforcing the time limit, everyone in the group will have an opportunity to participate. A common variation on this approach is the Think-Pair-Share where time is provided for individuals to develop a response prior to talking with their partner.

2. *Buzz groups:* This small group discussion technique is used to engage learners and re-energize the group. To initiate the buzz group, pose a question and ask learners to discuss their responses in pairs or groups no larger than four learners before sharing their work with the entire group. The room will soon be buzzing with conversation. This technique is useful for making a transition from one discussion task to another, or for encouraging learners to share ideas or concerns they might be reluctant to share with the entire group. As a small group teacher, your role is to facilitate the process and use the buzz group as a source of informal feedback about learners' understanding of the course material.

3. *Group round*: The purpose of this small group discussion technique is to involve everyone in the group and generate interest in a topic. Each learner provides a brief response, no more than 1 min, before moving on to the next learner. There are several ways to determine the order in which learners will participate. For consistency and efficiency, the teacher or group can determine the order at the beginning of the session. For a more spontaneous approach, the learner who is speaking can select the next learner, and this continues until all members of the group have participated. This method will generate more interest and engagement than the former two approaches. Learners may be permitted to pass at least one time during the group round.

4. *Brainstorming*: Brainstorming sessions are used to produce a large number of creative solutions or hypotheses in a short amount of time. This technique is also effective for encouraging learners to recall material learned at an earlier time. After a question or topic is identified, learners are asked to name ideas as they think of them. The group is forbidden to critique the ideas until after the brainstorming session has closed. Brainstorming promotes interaction within the group, but there are limitations to this strategy. For example, some learners may require more processing time to generate new ideas, and may not feel like they have much to contribute to the session until afterwards. Another potential problem is that some learners may choose not to participate. These "social loafers" may not have prepared sufficiently, and will gladly let others conduct the work of the group.

Table 3.2 Agenda for a role-playing session with two practice interviews

Activity
1. Attendance and announcements
2. Overview of the learning objectives and skills to be assessed during the interviewing session
3. Student 1 exits the room and waits for his/her interview
4. Student 2 interviews the standardized patient
5. The group provides feedback to student 2
6. Student 1 interviews the standardized patient
7. The group provides feedback to student 1
8. Wrap-up and review of key learning objectives

5. *Role-playing*: This strategy is particularly useful for learning and practicing communication skills such as interviewing or history taking. For some role-play sessions, it is possible to ask learners to play all of the roles (e.g., physician or patient) in the case or simulated encounter. For more advanced role-plays, including those that cover sensitive topics, it may be more appropriate to recruit and train standardized, actor patients. An example of an agenda for a role-playing session used in a course on interviewing skills is illustrated in Table 3.2.

Tools for Teaching and Learning in Small Groups

Tools such as Wi-Fi enabled tablets and smartphones; SMART™ boards; video; web-based reference materials; computer exercises; conferencing; and simulation can enhance small group learning and promote purposeful activity. Educational technologies have also made it easier for learners and teachers to communicate and share information outside of scheduled small group sessions. These technologies will be discussed in greater detail in Chap. 10, but it is worth noting that tools that create online communities, such as blogs, wikis, document sharing services and discussion boards, can be used to enhance the work of a face-to-face small group. For example, you might ask learners in your small group to maintain a blog and post brief reflections or questions after sessions that are particularly challenging. Unlike a traditional journal, the blog can include hyperlinks to other Web-based content, and can be accessed easily by others. Use caution, though, in assigning projects if they do not integrate into the course or students perceive their work on the assignments is not reviewed or acknowledged by you.

Evaluation of Small Group Participation and Learning

Evaluating small group participation and learning sends a message to learners that the activity is a meaningful part of the curriculum. Learners are also more likely to participate and prepare for the session if they know their contribution will count.

Criteria for assessing participation should be explicit. When possible, invite small group learners to participate in determining some of these criteria so they feel responsible for their learning and the success of the group. This should occur soon after the course begins, often at the time the group establishes rules and norms. Examples of criteria to assess participation include these expectations of the student:

- Contributes to the discussion with evidence of preparation.
- Provides comparative assessments.
- Builds upon others' contributions.
- Willing to listen to others.
- Respects different viewpoints.
- Provides constructive criticism.
- Helps to summarize the discussion.

Evaluation of Small Group Teaching

Teaching in small groups, like any teaching activity, will benefit from evaluation by learners and faculty. To evaluate your teaching, you will need to collect information that accurately describes the activity and then make a judgment about this information. Evaluation of teaching is discussed in greater detail in Chap. 16, but a few points specific to teaching in small groups merit attention here.

Formative Evaluation

Informal, formative evaluation can be useful for identifying aspects of the small group experience that detract from learning but can be corrected while the course is still in session. Examples of methods to collect informal evaluation data include brief online surveys; fast feedback cards collected at the end of a session; and periodic group debriefings.

Summative Evaluation

Summative, or formal, evaluation of small group teaching should draw upon multiple sources of data and seek to promote validity and reliability. One source of data is student evaluations or questionnaires. Most departments or schools provide these, and items typically address topics such as the small group instructor's ability to facilitate the group, contribution of small group activities to improving understanding of the material, quality of resource materials, workload or amount of material covered, organization of the small group activities, and feedback on learning. Peer review of teaching is another source of valuable data. Colleagues who are knowledgeable about the subject can observe and evaluate how well the small group sessions promote discussion and understanding of key concepts. Colleagues who are not content experts can provide helpful insight into group dynamics and your skills as a facilitator. If your school does not provide resources for peer review of teaching, consult Chism's (2007) comprehensive guide to peer review of teaching. This includes resources and observation forms to ensure standardized assessment. A third source of data is video recordings of small group sessions. Some small group instructors find it helpful to review recordings, sometimes with the assistance of an educational consultant or trusted colleague, to identify aspects of teaching that require improvement. While all of these methods can provide useful data, be careful to ensure reliability by examining your teaching on multiple occasions. The interactive and personal nature of small group teaching makes it rewarding, but also highly variable.

References

Anderson LW, Krathwohl DR (eds), Airasian PW, Cruikshank KA, Mayer RE, Pintrich PR, Raths J, Wittrock MC (2001) A taxonomy for learning, teaching, and assessing: a revision of Bloom's taxonomy of educational objectives (Complete edition). Longman, New York

Chism N (2007) Peer review of teaching. Anker Publishing Co, Bolton

Engelhart MD, Furst EJ, Hill WH, Krathwohl DR (1956) Taxonomy of educational objectives: the classification of educational goals. In: Bloom BS (ed) Handbook 1: cognitive domain. David McKay, New York

Jacques D (2003) Teaching small groups. BMJ 326:492–494

Keirsey D (1998) Please understand me II: temperament, character, intelligence. Prometheus Nemesis Book Company, Del Mar

Kolb DA (1984) Experiential learning: experience as the source of learning and development. Prentice-Hall, Englewood Cliffs

Myers IB, Myers PB (1995) Gifts differing: understanding personality type. Davies-Black Publishing, Mountain View

Newble D, Cannon R (2001) A handbook for medical teachers, 4th edn. Kluwer Academic Publishers, Dordrecht

Scholtes PR, Joiner BL, Joiner BJ (2000) The TEAM handbook. Oriel, Inc, Madison

Steinert Y (2004) Student perceptions of effective small group teaching. Med Educ 38:286–293

Stiggins RJ, Rubel E, Quellmalz E (1988) Measuring thinking skills in the classroom, rev ed. National Education Assn Professional Library, West Haven

Tuckman B (1965) Developmental sequence in small groups. Psychol Bull 63:384–399

Westberg J, Jason H (1996) Fostering learning in small groups: a practical guide. Springer, New York

For Further Reading

For a concise summary of recommendations for teaching in small groups, review Jacques D (2003) ABC of teaching and learning in medicine: Teaching small groups. Br Med J 326:492–494

For an in-depth examination of the concepts and techniques introduced in this chapter, consult Westberg J, Jason H (1996) Fostering learning in small groups: a practical guide. Springer, New York

For further reading on the conditions for establishing effective small groups, read Wlodkowski RJ (1999) Enhancing adult motivation to learn. Jossey-Bass, San Francisco, CA

Chapter 4
Flipping the Classroom

William B. Jeffries and Kathryn N. Huggett

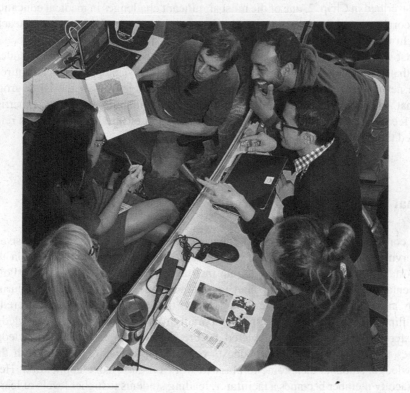

W.B. Jeffries, Ph.D. (✉)
Office of Medical Education, University of Vermont College of Medicine,
The Courtyard at Given, N117, 89 Beaumont Ave, Burlington, VT 05405, USA
e-mail: wbjeffri@uvm.edu

K.N. Huggett, Ph.D.
Office of Medical Education, Creighton University School of Medicine,
2500 California Plaza, Criss III, Room 463, Omaha, NE 68178, USA
e-mail: kathrynhuggett@creighton.edu

K.N. Huggett and W.B. Jeffries (eds.), *An Introduction to Medical Teaching*,
DOI 10.1007/978-94-017-9066-6_4, © Springer Science+Business Media Dordrecht 2014

Abstract In this chapter, we discuss a new movement among educators that goes beyond simply enhancing lectures. Here the lecture is replaced entirely with new types of learning, while preserving the efficiencies of the large group format. In this model, the aim is to maximize the availability of faculty expertise and feedback, take advantage of group learning, and ensure that learning is reinforced through application rather than memorization. This chapter details how to prepare, implement and troubleshoot a "flipped" classroom through a variety of customizable strategies.

Introduction

As described in Chap. 2, one of the most significant challenges in medical education is incorporating active learning in an environment dominated by large group teaching. In that chapter, methods for incorporation of active learning *into* the lecture format were discussed. In this chapter, we discuss a new movement among educators that goes beyond simply enhancing lectures. Here the lecture is replaced entirely with new types of learning, while preserving the efficiencies of the large group format. In this model, the aim is to maximize the availability of faculty expertise and feedback, take advantage of group learning, and ensure that learning is reinforced through application rather than memorization.

What Is the "Flipped Classroom?"

In a conventional lecture format, the learner obtains knowledge by: (1) passively observing a performance by an expert faculty member, (2) taking notes on the important points and (3) referring to an instructor-provided outline or PowerPoint presentation. This experience is later recounted in the student's own mind during study and during homework, i.e., assignments that must be completed for credit. The flipped classroom model turns this paradigm inside out. Here the knowledge transfer *is* the homework, completed before coming to class. This knowledge comes from assigned reading, podcasts or video of a lecture. Armed with this knowledge, students then come to class to work on knowledge application. Here the faculty member becomes a facilitator, leading students to higher levels of learning and retention. The desired result is higher levels of learning and engagement, optimization of faulty time and the ability to expand learning objectives to domains outside of knowledge acquisition (e.g., professionalism, communication skills, critical thinking). Most importantly, students have ready access to expert help (you) and peer teaching as they attempt to apply their newly acquired knowledge to real world problems.

Principles of the Flipped Classroom

The primary purpose of the flipped classroom is to remove simple knowledge acquisition from the classroom setting and to reserve classroom time for knowledge application and clarification. To achieve this aim, the following principles can effectively guide the design and execution of a successful flipped classroom experience:

- Students must have clear objectives for knowledge acquisition and access to materials that succinctly provide them with this information.
- The sources of assigned knowledge acquisition must be concise and focused to allow students to complete it before attending class.
- Students learn best in context; thus assigned class work should be focused on significant problems requiring application of their new knowledge and higher levels of learning.
- Peer teaching magnifies learning; thus assigned classwork is best designed for and conducted in groups.
- Assessment drives learning; thus assessment of class performance is desired and course assessments should mirror the higher level learning that has occurred in class, not merely the knowledge acquired in pre-class work.

An important outcome of the flipped classroom is the ability to achieve higher levels of learning inside the classroom. This can be understood by considering the progression of learning through a formally identified framework of learning objectives. A group of educators chaired by Benjamin Bloom (1956) originally defined a taxonomy of six types of cognitive learning objectives that increase in complexity that can be conceptualized in the form of a pyramid. This progression from bottom to top includes the recall of facts, patterns, and concepts important for developing the cognitive domain of learning (i.e., intellectual abilities and skills). Individuals usually master one level before progressing to the next. A modified version (Krathwohl 2002, Schultz 2005) is shown below:

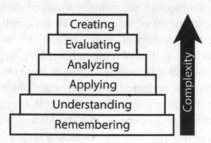

Importantly, in the traditional lecture format, students participate with little preparation. Learning therefore begins at the bottom of the pyramid. Mastery of the Remembering and Understanding levels is attempted during the lecture. Unfortunately, even this is difficult in lecture since students have not yet had time to assimilate the material and are subject to the loss of attention described in Chap. 2. Further, since students have varying abilities, there will be wide gaps in student understanding at the completion of the lecture. If the student has difficulty with lower levels of understanding, there is little opportunity to address that formally through in-class instructor intervention or peer teaching. Higher levels of learning await solitary homework assignments that may challenge student understanding and stimulate student understanding. Instructor feedback and peer teaching is not optimized in the traditional lecture format.

In flipped classroom approaches, students are expected to progress through the first two levels of Bloom's Taxonomy and begin work on mastering application and beyond. Ideal assignments are designed to stimulate recall and understanding by requiring students to *do* something with the knowledge they have acquired. Gaps in understanding are filled with peer teaching and instructor feedback. This allows for students to catch up and achieve similar levels of learning at the conclusion of the session. It also allows a higher level of assessment to take place as test questions can cover student reasoning and not simple recall.

Since efficiency and increased depth of learning are important goals of the flipped classroom it is important to consider the optimal ways to structure and execute the components of the flipped classroom. These include the pre-classroom activities, the flipped session, and assessment.

Pre-classroom Activities: Turning Your Lecture into Homework

Careful consideration is required when replacing lectures with flipped sessions. First and foremost, students must have clear objectives for the session as they approach their preparatory assignments. These objectives should be constructed using verbs associated with the new Bloom's taxonomy that **describe what the student will be able to do at the end of the session**. This way, students can prepare in a focused manner and not waste time guessing what will be covered. For example, if the topic is the treatment of the complications of diabetes and the reading assignment includes the treatment of diabetes AND its complications, students will react strongly about the time spent over-preparing and they will lack enthusiasm in the flipped session. Thus having clear objectives provides a map for student preparation and a map for the instructor to understand what students should be able to do by the end of the session. It is preferred to have distinct objectives for the preparatory assignment and the flipped classroom experience. In the case of the preparatory assignment, the instructor usually expects that the learner will accomplish objectives that relate to the remembering and understanding stages of Bloom's taxonomy. Objectives covering the higher stages will be addressed in the classroom.

The knowledge acquisition assignment must be focused and reasonable with respect to time needed for completion. This can be accomplished through reading assignments, specific handouts created for the topic, podcasts of previous lectures, new lectures created for the flipped session or videos from other sources (e.g., YouTube). A combination of any of these can be employed as long as the standard of reasonable workload is maintained and they are relevant to the session objectives

(Saltman 2011). If assigning readings, it is helpful to identify succinct sources such as review articles or textbook chapters. Some instructors make handouts with specific excerpts that are most relevant to learning (ensure the copyright provisions are respected!). It is also helpful to construct short formative quizzes on fact recall or understanding that students can take online to ensure their readiness. As discussed below, these quizzes could be reserved for the beginning of the flipped session to ensure attendance and improve readiness.

It is common for faculty to assign podcasts as the preparatory assignment. When choosing this route, several considerations come to mind. Faculty members are tempted to use podcasts of old lectures as the knowledge assignment, since they are usually assured of completeness of content coverage and are confident that the student got at least as much material covered as they did before the introduction of the flipped classroom. We strongly discourage this approach. Captured lectures are subject to many of the problems that were discussed in Chap. 2 (e.g., loss of attention). The sheer length of the sessions makes them ripe for loss of engagement. In addition, captured lectures include many irrelevant moments that are not conducive to a preparatory session: pauses and gaps as the instructor reiterates previously learned concepts and answers student questions, jokes and (hopefully) active learning components intended for a live audience. A better approach is to create specific video podcasts for each session that are short (about 10 min) and succinct, covering the material in a narrated slideshow or virtual chalk-talk. Such an approach was recently suggested by Prober and Khan (2013). This approach allows students to break down concepts into easily understood components, review the videos if needed and complete the work in their own time. These authors also stress the incorporation of only "evergreen" material, i.e., material that is foundational and highly likely to be true (as opposed to controversial or still experimental data). Controversy and experimental data can serve however, as learning tools for the flipped session to climb the pyramid of Bloom's taxonomy.

Flipped Classroom Preparation

Setting Up the Room

The physical setting for the flipped classroom is likely the same room where you have conducted your lectures. Ideally this would be in a room with a flat floor, with tables and movable chairs to allow students to configure themselves into learning groups. Often, the flipped session must take place in a tiered classroom that is better suited for viewing a lecture than participating in a group activity. This can inhibit, but not prevent, an effective flipped classroom exercise. Students should be encouraged to assume configurations that work best for them in a group learning situation. Group size can vary from two to six or seven, depending on the exercise, so keep the room layout in mind when configuring the session. Acoustics are important, and expect an active learning classroom to be loud during discussions but quiet when students are called upon to address the class from their places.

Design of the Session

One of the best features of designing a flipped learning experience is that there are many types of activities that can be employed to hold student interest and contribute to learning. Prior to beginning the activity, one should ask several relevant questions:

- Assuming that students have met the knowledge objectives in the preparatory session, what will you expect the students to do with that information? This forms the basis for writing the session objectives.
- How will you to assure readiness and participation? Students who do not complete the assigned work will not be effective participants in classroom work, so an effective session must deal with this question.
- What activities will be used and how will they be applied toward meeting the objectives? In the next section, a variety of possible activities are introduced that can be used to stimulate individual or group learning.
- How will learning be assessed? Assessment of learning plays an important part in the design of the session. Holding students accountable for advanced stages of their learning is essential to making the flipped classroom successful.

Readiness Assurance

Readiness assurance is a term borrowed from Team-Based Learning (Chap. 6). If students do not prepare for the session, it is doomed to failure since they have not considered, much less mastered the lower level objectives. This can lead to failure in meeting the upper objectives and poor attendance. To prevent this, many adherents either require participation through mandatory attendance policies or have participation in some way count toward the student grade. The easiest way to accomplish this is to administer a quiz at the beginning of the session. The quiz should ideally be short, address the objectives of the preparatory session and should contribute to the final course grade. This ensures that students take the assignment seriously and present themselves ready to learn. Other ways include completion of online assessments or assignments prior to participation in an online bulletin board, Wiki, etc. It is also possible to use peer assessment to ensure that students police whether students in their study group are dutifully preparing for the flipped classroom.

The Flipped Classroom Session

There are innumerable ways to design a flipped classroom session, and we will present two major categories here, "Homework in Class" and "Classroom Assessment Techniques."

Homework in Class and Related Techniques

Worksheet

This is the simplest (and least engaging) of flipped classroom sessions. Lecturers have often provided worksheets to students to practice application of discussed concepts (e.g., mathematics problems, chemical reactions, etc.). Sheets are returned to the instructor for grading as a homework assignment. In the flipped setting, the classroom becomes the venue for filling out a worksheet based on assigned activities (readings, podcasts, videos, etc.).

Suggestions for Application

1. Do not make this the entire session, as students get bored fairly quickly.
2. Distribute the worksheet during class – if you hand it out in advance (or if students have access to it from previous students), students will avoid the session.
3. Allow students to complete it as a group. This allows students with a better grasp of the material to teach those who need help.
4. Combine the worksheet with adapted classroom assessment techniques (see below) to maximize the benefit.
5. Allow each group to submit one worksheet for credit, or give a short quiz at the end of the session containing similar problems to ensure that all students have achieved session objectives.

Dry Lab

A common practice among medical science educators is to provide students with the opportunity to design experiments and/or interpret provided laboratory data based on concepts presented in lecture. Results can be returned to the instructor for grading. In the flipped classroom, knowledge objectives are assigned and satisfied outside of lecture (e.g., assigned readings, podcasts, videos) and the "dry lab" occupies the space formerly used for the lecture. Students or groups of students can be called upon to present the results near the end of the session.

Suggestions for Application

1. Distribute the dry lab data during class – if you hand it out in advance (or if students have access to it from previous students), students will avoid the session.
2. Have students work in small groups to complete assigned labs. Weaker students can be helped by peer teaching from stronger students. Faculty can "float" and answer difficult questions (but NOT lecture!).
3. Have students submit completed group work before presentations to ensure everyone participates.

4. Vary lab material from year to year to ensure students won't use material and answers from previously enrolled students.
5. Assess achievement of objectives with a short set of relevant problems at the end of, or shortly after the session.

Case Report

A common practice among medical science educators is to provide students with a case report scenario, slowly revealing aspects of the case as they unfold chronologically. The case can be on paper or involve a standardized or simulated patient. This format is often used in small groups, based on didactic material from the curriculum. This can easily be flipped to a large group session. Many of the concepts discussed for "dry lab" apply here. If knowledge objectives are assigned and satisfied outside of lecture (e.g., assigned readings, podcasts, videos) the case report can occupy the space formerly used for the lecture.

Suggestions for Application

1. Provide some details of the case before class to encourage focused reading. We do not recommend giving out specific questions before class, except for one or two standard questions that go with EVERY case that have been developed so that students can orient themselves. If you hand out all material in advance (or if student have access to it from previous students), students will either avoid the session or deliver the answers in rote fashion.
2. Have students work in small groups to complete case questions. Cases can be done in episodes with large group discussion following small group deliberation, or cases can be worked out in small groups in their entirety. Weaker students can be helped by peer teaching from stronger students. Faculty can "float" and answer difficult questions (but NOT lecture!).
3. Students could develop a case note in SOAP or some other standard format as an in-class product. The SOAP note could then be used for a case presentation by selected students/groups.
4. Have students submit completed group work before presentations to ensure everyone participates.
5. Vary cases material from year to year to ensure students won't use material and answers from previously enrolled students.
6. Assess achievement of objectives with a short set of relevant problems at the end or shortly after the session.

Review Session

Instructors or course directors sometimes include scheduled review sessions before exams to ensure students can bring their questions regarding the course material to faculty. In the flipped classroom, if students have achieved knowledge objectives without attending lecture, all or part of a scheduled lecture time can be devoted to answering students' questions.

Suggestions for Application

1. Avoid being drawn into giving a "mini-lecture." Students must be prepared to ask specific questions and the instructor must resist the desire to facilitate passive learning methods.
2. A review session is best combined with or replaced by classroom assessment techniques to ensure maximum participation and learning.

Adapted Classroom Assessment Techniques

Angelo and Cross (1993) compiled a number of effective ways to introduce active learning into an otherwise passive lecture (see examples in Chap. 2). Since the intent of these techniques was to engage students and promote higher order learning, it is relatively easy to envision how to adapt them to a flipped classroom. Some of these methods are presented below, but the reader is urged to consult the original literature to discover other classroom assessment techniques that could be of use in the flipped environment.

Background Knowledge Probe

The background knowledge probe is designed to determine student's prior knowledge, their recall and understanding of material key to success in a course or unit. The probe is usually in the form of a multiple choice or short answer test. In a flipped classroom, students can be assigned one or more prior readings, podcasts or videos to gain subject knowledge. The large group class meeting can then begin with an assessment that can be taken individually or in groups (or in the case of Team Based Learning, both).

Suggestions for Application

1. Use this to start a session
2. In multiple choice format, an audience response system can be used by the instructor to quickly gauge student understanding of key concepts.
3. Short answer format can be effective for recall not based on word recognition. The probe can be graded quickly by neighboring students.
4. The exam can be used as a tool to encourage group learning and peer teaching. In Team-Based Learning, students complete initial assessments alone and then complete the same exam within a small group. This enables students to help each other clarify unclear points for each other and stimulates all students to participate in application of their knowledge.
5. Students take the exercise much more seriously if the assessment counts toward their grade.

The One-Minute Paper

The one-minute paper is used to assess prior knowledge, recall and understanding of key concepts. Traditionally, it can be used at the beginning or at any point during class when an important concept needs to be emphasized and imprinted into long-term memory. The paper is often in response to a question like "what is the most salient feature of the process we discussed today" or "what concepts covered today are key to the treatment of X disease," etc. The papers are graded and returned to students at the next session. For a flipped session, students can be tasked to either summarize the key concepts derived from class preparation (e.g., reading, podcast, video) or can summarize portions of a group discussion related to the application of a topic during the flipped classroom session.

Suggestions for Application

1. Can be used to start a session, or at any time during the active session.
2. The essay can be handed in for credit or graded by neighboring student to stimulate discussion.
3. Students can be called on to read their short essays, to stimulate discussion.
4. Students can be assigned to develop an essay together, based on an assigned discussion or problem set that draws on their knowledge.
5. A variation involves groups of students creating a presentation during a learning session that summarizes key points. The presentation can be delivered near the end of the session or posted or podcast for further use by all students. The faculty challenge is to ensure expectations of accuracy and presentation quality.
6. Students take the exercise much more seriously if the assessment counts toward their grade.

The Muddiest Point

The muddiest point is a technique whereby students quickly note the greatest area(s) of difficulty ("the muddiest point") that they have with lecture material or assigned readings. In a lecture setting this is compiled at the end of class and the teacher returns in the following session to clarify the most frequent difficulties. In the flipped classroom, students can be given the routine assignment of specifying the muddiest point from assigned material and bringing those questions to the active session. If bringing a muddy point to class is required, it improves engagement and preparation.

Suggestions for Application

1. Best used in the middle or at the end of the session ("muddy points" can sometimes develop into lengthy diversions!)
2. The question can be introduced into a small group formed among neighbors (or to pre-assigned groups) to stimulate discussion and peer teaching

3. Difficult questions not solved by the group can be presented to the larger group for resolution. Resist the temptation to break into a spontaneous lecture in response to a muddy point – peer discussion is better.
4. Students can be assigned to develop a group response that summarizes key points. The response can be presented near the end of the session or posted or podcast for further use by all students. The faculty challenge is to ensure expectations of accuracy and presentation quality.
5. Students take the exercise much more seriously if the assessment counts toward their grade.

The One-Sentence Summary

In the original lecture format, the instructor asks each student to prepare a declarative sentence that summarizes a key point. This works well when summarizing factual information such as pathways or reasoning paradigms (e.g., "When assessing hyponatremia one must first ascertain volume status…"). In the flipped classroom, the instructor asks the learners to develop one sentence summaries for specific topics that they can look up or develop from recalled knowledge or from the active session. If bringing a one sentence summary to class is required, it improves engagement and preparation.

Suggestions for Application

1. Can be used to summarize prepared or discussed material.
2. Can be the result of a group small group discussion formed among neighbors to stimulate discussion and peer teaching.
3. Students can be assigned to develop a group sentence that summarizes a key point. The sentence can be presented near the end of the session or posted or podcast for further use by all students. The faculty challenge is to ensure expectations of accuracy and presentation quality.
4. Sentences from different students/groups on similar topics can be read aloud and students can vote on the best ones using an audience response system.
5. Students take the exercise much more seriously if the assessment counts toward their grade.

Directed Paraphrasing

This method requires students to paraphrase a specific part of a lesson in their own words. This makes the learner directly apply and present their newly acquired knowledge and reasoning skills. In the flipped setting, students can be asked to take a small amount of time to summarize a portion of an assigned lesson or repeat key points from the discussion. The latter aspect of this is already in routine use in clerkship presentations of patients on rounds.

Suggestions for Application

1. Can be used to summarize prepared or discussed material.
2. Students can be called on to summarize for an assembled peer group the key points of the assignment. DANGER: students could internally assign the task of preparing for the session on a rotating basis, thus eliminating the need for all students to prepare for the session.
3. The best use of this technique is to assign students to work on a specific problem or case, then have one of them summarize the findings for the large group.
4. Students can be assessed on their participation and presentation skills, as well as content knowledge. Peers can participate in the assessment process.

Application Cards

After learning a concept, students are given a card to write down possible real world applications of this knowledge. Cards are assessed on a Likert scale with feedback. In a flipped classroom, students can understand basic science concepts and their relevance better when presented in the context of clinical medicine. Thus, assigned preparation material can be more readily understood if students are expected to relate it to a relevant disease process, or wellness concept. Students can be asked to produce a short written description of the application of a particular basic science topic.

Suggestions for Application

1. Can be used for prepared or discussed material.
2. Students can be assigned the task of developing individual, non-overlapping cards based on key discussion points. The instructor can then call for unique applications from selected groups.
3. Cards from different students/groups on similar topics can be read aloud and students can vote on the best ones using an audience response system.
4. Students take the exercise much more seriously if the assessment counts toward their grade.

Student-Generated Test Questions

Students are asked to develop several exam questions with one best answer. This method develops comprehension and application skills. In a flipped classroom, learners can be assigned the task of preparing exam questions based on assigned material or developing them in class. Caution: since many students use commercially available question banks for their studies, plagiarism is a concern. Students generally prefer preparing for exams by using practice questions, so this method can be very popular.

Suggestions for Application

1. Students should be oriented to the principles of valid examination formats and question styles.
2. Students could be assigned the task of individually generating three exam questions. Working in groups students discuss the questions and attempt to modify and merge their group's question pool into a comprehensive ten-question quiz.
3. Generated (and accurate) questions can be posted on a student bulletin board or other suitable venue for their study.
4. Students could be further motivated by the promised use of a small number of their questions on the actual exam.

Pro and Con Grid

Learners are asked to chart the pros and cons of a specific issue or topic, which is useful in developing and assessing critical thinking skills. Students can be asked to develop a chart of the pros and cons regarding ethical or risk/benefit of certain treatments or public health approaches to societal problems, etc.

Suggestions for Application

1. Students can be assigned to apply assigned knowledge objectives to real world problems before coming to class. Students can work in groups to discuss specific cases and discuss to refine their grids.
2. Grids can be developed by individual groups, and presented for large group discussion, comparing and contrasting the work of individual groups. A consensus grid can be developed for the entire class and posted online for later assessment.

A Final Word

Assessment of Student Progress

Readiness assurance activities promote self-assessment and accountability and In-class application activities also constitute formative assessment in the flipped classroom session. The true determination of effectiveness of the flipped classroom experience is the lasting educational outcome. This will come in the course assessments, subsequent performance in later courses and clerkships, and application of acquired knowledge and skills in clinical practice. It is important to remember to align the learning and formative assessment activities in class with the course objectives and summative course assessments. What you choose to measure on assessments sends a powerful message to students and they will detect if a mismatch in rigor is present between classroom activities and questions on course examinations. Thus you should ensure that summative course assessments include higher order questions and not just knowledge recall questions. This will reinforce learning and provide an immediate reward for students who seek to maximize the effectiveness of active learning.

Troubleshooting the Active Learning Setting

Active learning exercises are subject to unexpected turns that may derail even the best planning. It is important to remain flexible and be willing and able to change class activities as needed. These disruptions can come in many forms. The physical environment may be disrupted (fire alarm, technology failure, etc.). Develop class norms or guidelines that are agreed to in advance that can handle contingencies in case of such disruptions. A social contract can also be developed with learners to handle classroom behavior. Students who don't prepare are often the biggest problem: It is best to let this be handled by peers in the group (either through explicit rules or peer assessment), or use for credit in-class assessments to address lack of preparation and participation. A final difficulty may be colleagues who agree to facilitate but appear to give mini-lectures as they circulate around the room. Be prepared to redirect these peers before they undermine the intended activity. Gently remind them that the students should be asking the questions of each other.

Barriers to Implementation

The primary barrier is your own imagination. Creative planning can overcome most barriers, but time is needed to plan challenging in-class activities. Do not attempt to "wing it" as some of the aforementioned difficulties can prevent effective implementation. Attempt to secure an optimal room size and layout for the flipped classroom, in which students can effectively collaborate. If only a tiered classroom is available, it is effective to group students with those directly behind them. As mentioned previously, the assignment materials should be judiciously distributed to prevent some students from undermining flipped classroom learning activities. In our experience, if students have all the learning materials in advance, some will strategically assign completion of the work in advance of sessions. These students may perform well on the formative assessments, but the collaborative, discovery-based learning process will be stunted when everyone knows the answers in advance.

It is clear that the flipped classroom provides an excellent opportunity to energize the classroom by engaging students and faculty in an effective way to stimulate learning. We anticipate that as the use of this modality grows, that many more innovations will be introduced to create an even more dynamic way of teaching.

References

Angelo TA, Cross KP (1993) Classroom assessment techniques: a handbook for college teachers. Jossey-Bass, San Francisco

Engelhart MD, Furst EJ, Hill WH, Krathwohl DR (1956) Taxonomy of educational objectives: the classification of educational goals. In: Bloom BS (ed) Handbook 1: cognitive domain. David McKay, New York

Krathwohl DR (2002) A revision of Bloom's taxonomy: an overview. Theory Pract 41(4): 212–218. At http://dx.doi.org/10.1207/s15430421tip4104_2. Accessed 5 Mar 2014

Prober CG, Khan S (2013) Medical education reimagined: a call to action. Acad Med 88(10):1407–1410

Saltman D (2011) Flipping for beginners; inside the new classroom craze. Harv Educ Lett 27(6). http://www.hepg.org/hel/article/517. Accessed 5 Mar 2014

Schultz L (2005) Lynn Schultz: Old Dominion University: Bloom's taxonomy. Retrieved March 5, 2014, from http://ww2.odu.edu/educ/roverbau/Bloom/blooms_taxonomy.htm

For Further Reading

For a detailed "how to" website of flipping the classroom, review the Center for Teaching and Learning at Vanderbilt University: http://cft.vanderbilt.edu/guides-sub-pages/flipping-the-classroom/. Accessed 5 Mar 2014

A website maintained by Jerry Overmyer showing how to use screencasting to "flip" the classroom. Flipping the classroom: educational vodcasting. http://www.flippedclassroom.com. Accessed 5 Mar 2014

For an example on how a Pharmacy program flipped their Pharmaceutics course to enhance student learning. See McLaughlin JE, Roth MT, Glatt DM, Gharkholonarehe N, Davidson CA, Griffin LM, Esserman DA, Mumper RJ (2014) The flipped classroom: a course redesign to foster learning and engagement in a health professions school. Acad Med 89(2):236–243

Chapter 5
Problem-Based Learning

Mark A. Albanese and Laura C. Dast

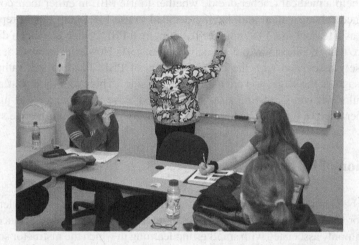

Abstract Problem-based learning (PBL) was created at McMaster University almost 40 years ago. It has changed medical education in ways that would not have been foreseen. It has supplanted the traditional lecture-based learning model in many medical schools and has expanded around the world and beyond medical education into a host of other disciplines. It has also galvanized the push to get students out of the lecture hall and into more interactive learning settings. This chapter is designed with two purposes in mind: to help a medical teacher decide whether to use PBL in

M.A. Albanese, Ph.D. (✉)
Professor Emeritus, Departments of Population Health Sciences
and Educational Psychology, School of Medicine and Public Health
and College of Education, University of Wisconsin-Madison,
610 Walnut Street, 1007C Madison, Wisconsin 53726-2397, USA
e-mail: maalbane@wisc.edu

L.C. Dast
School of Medicine and Public Health, University of Wisconsin, Madison, WI, USA

K.N. Huggett and W.B. Jeffries (eds.), *An Introduction to Medical Teaching*,
DOI 10.1007/978-94-017-9066-6_5, © Springer Science+Business Media Dordrecht 2014

either their course or broader medical curriculum and, having decided to use PBL, help them prepare for their role as a teacher in a PBL course. Teaching in a PBL course is a much different experience than in almost any other teaching format.

Introduction

Problem-based learning (PBL) was created at McMaster University over 40 years ago. It has changed medical education in ways that would not have been foreseen. It has supplanted the traditional lecture-based learning model in many medical schools and has expanded around the world and beyond medical education into a host of other disciplines. It has also galvanized the push to get students out of the lecture hall and into more interactive learning settings. This chapter is designed with two purposes in mind: to help a medical teacher decide whether to use PBL in either their course or broader medical curriculum and, having decided to use PBL, help them prepare for their role as a teacher in a PBL course. Teaching in a PBL course is a much different experience than in almost any other teaching format. As Howard Barrows, the person most closely associated with the broad adoption of PBL, liked to say, rather than "being a sage on the stage, you are a guide on the side." This takes some getting used to, particularly if you like being a sage and/or you crave the stage, or you just have never experienced a form of teaching where you were not THE authoritative source.

Definition of PBL

PBL can be characterized as an instructional method that uses patient problems as a context for students to acquire knowledge about the basic and clinical sciences. It is most commonly associated with small group learning in which the instructor serves as a facilitator. As a facilitator, the instructor's role is to ensure that the process of PBL is carried out, not to dispense knowledge. The process of PBL is to place the focus on the students and to allow them free inquiry into how to solve the problem. Specifically, the facilitator has three tasks: to help students organize their group to function effectively, to ensure that all members of the group have an opportunity to participate fully, and to adjust their course if they deviate too far from the desired path. Originally, PBL was designed to be an overarching curriculum that required a major reallocation of time allotted to various educational activities. After the time for structured activities was reduced, there was a major restructuring in how the remaining required time was allocated to lecture, small group, lab, etc. A number of medical schools maintain two curriculum tracks, one traditional lecture-based and the other PBL. In recent years, there has been a trend for schools that have dual tracks to merge them into one, adopting the best of both curricula into a single combined "hybrid" curriculum. There have also been efforts to institute PBL in individual courses embedded within curricula that employed largely lecture-based learning methods.

Research on the effectiveness of PBL has been somewhat disappointing to those who expected PBL to be a radical improvement in medical education. Several reviews of PBL over the past 20 years have not shown the gains in performance that many had hoped for; such studies have been limited by design weaknesses inherent in evaluating curricula. While the research indicates that PBL curricula have not produced graduates who are demonstrably inferior to graduates of other types of curricula; whether they are superior is an open question. There is some evidence that students from a PBL curriculum function better in clinically related activities and students and faculty consistently report enjoying learning and teaching in a PBL format. However, there has been concern expressed that students in a PBL curriculum may develop less complete cognitive scaffolding for basic science material. This may relate to the somewhat disconcerting trend that approximately 5–10 % of students do not do well in a PBL curriculum. If able these students often change tracks after having difficulty in the PBL track. However, as schools have merged tracks into hybrid curricula, this trend has become less evident.

Introducing PBL into the Curriculum

The challenges likely to be encountered in implementing PBL depend to a large degree upon the scope of implementation that is being considered. If it is a change in the entire medical curriculum, it will be a much different process than if a course director is deciding whether to implement it in his/her course. In either case, a review of the evidence for and against PBL would be an important first step. The gains that are hoped for will need to be weighed against the cost to make the change. The arguments used for changing to PBL will be more compelling if they are buttressed by evidence. This will be especially important if the change is to be curriculum-wide as opposed to a single course. Since 1990, there have been at least 20 major reviews. Somewhat surprisingly, the three published in 1993 still have currency. Vernon and Blake (1993) reported a meta-analysis of controlled trials, Albanese and Mitchell (1993) reported what might be considered a best evidence synthesis and Berkson (1993) conducted a thematic review. There have been more recent reports in the literature that postulate that a large degree of change should be expected from PBL to offer sufficient evidence (Colliver 2000; Cohen 1988). While the outcomes have not been overwhelmingly different for PBL, what may give PBL an edge over lecture-based learning is the ability to exercise greater control over the content and information density of the curriculum. Adding a lecture or making an existing lecture more dense (curriculum creep) can be done with little or no fanfare in a lecture-based curriculum. In contrast, increasing the number of problems or changing the nature of a problem to make it more information dense would demand careful consideration by PBL curriculum managers. The added scrutiny that changes demand in a PBL curriculum puts a damper on curriculum creep.

If you wish to implement PBL in your class, you should consider how to do this within the larger curriculum and the physical space and teaching constraints. Students need to have the ability to meet together in small groups with a facilitator and have access to information resources. Implementation in a course is also challenging because the types of problems that take the fullest advantage of the PBL structure tend to be multidisciplinary. The ideal situation is to have dedicated space for each small group that is equipped with technical support that allows internet access, electronic capture of white-board writing, and refreshments. However, this level of support is unlikely to be feasible in a single class use of PBL and the logistics of using multidisciplinary cases in a single course can be extremely difficult to manage. However, with some creativity and relaxing of the generally accepted requirements, it has been done (see Farrell et al. 1999).

Implementation across the entire medical school curriculum takes substantial effort. In schools that have made a major shift to PBL, the impetus or at least unquestioned support of the medical school Dean has been a driving force. There are resource allocation issues for space, faculty salary support and technical support that make any such implementation without the Dean's full support virtually impossible. Consensus among faculty is critical to begin implementation. The evidence and reviews cited earlier have been helpful to the governing bodies that have made such decisions. New medical schools have had the most success in starting PBL curricula (e.g., McMaster, Florida State University). There have been cases where whole medical school curricula have been converted to PBL, examples include the University of Iowa College of Medicine, Sherbrooke University, and the University of Missouri-Columbia. More commonly, schools have adopted a PBL track, in which admission is competitive and only a fraction of the entire class who volunteer and apply for the PBL track are admitted. Examples of this approach include Southern Illinois University, University of New Mexico, Harvard University and Michigan State University. The advantages of adopting a track approach are that it does not require a commitment from all faculty, small groups can usually be accommodated more easily, the value and feasibility of PBL can be demonstrated for those who have doubts, and all of the "bugs" in the PBL system can be worked out in a more controlled manner. In many cases, schools that began by adopting a track have eventually merged the PBL and traditional tracks into a hybrid that looks more like PBL than the traditional lecture-based learning curriculum.

Curriculum and Course Design

According to Barrows (1985), PBL is most compatible with an organ-based curriculum, in which courses are aligned with different organs of the body. Thus, a course on the cardiovascular system would have the anatomy, physiology, biochemistry, etc. of the cardiovascular system all integrated. Because patient problems are often localized to a single organ system, it seems logical that PBL would be consistent with an organ-based curriculum. For a course embedded in a lecture-based learning curriculum, those courses that are clinically focused are most compatible with a PBL format. In this type of curriculum, adopting PBL in basic science courses such as biochemistry or physiology will be more difficult due to the limited focus of the course. Integrating concepts that are the focus of other courses into the PBL cases of your course can be challenging to coordinate at the very least.

PBL Definitions

Before going into the larger issues of how to support PBL course design, it will be helpful to give a more specific definition of what has been considered the prototype PBL process (reiterative PBL in Barrow's taxonomy, 1986).

1. The process begins with a patient problem. Resources accompanying the problem include detailed objectives, print materials, audiovisual resources, multiple choice self-assessment exercises and resource faculty.
2. Students work in small groups, sometimes called tutorial groups; 6–8 students per group is often recommended.
3. The small groups are moderated by one or more faculty facilitators (sometimes called tutors, I prefer to use the term facilitator because a tutor to me is someone with content expertise that is trying to individually teach a student).
4. Students determine their own learning needs to address the problem, make assignments to each other to obtain needed information and then return to report what they have learned and continue with the problem. This happens repeatedly as students secure more information and keep probing deeper into the problem.
5. Students return for a final debriefing and analyze the approach they took after getting feedback on their case report.
6. Student evaluation occurs in a small group session and is derived from input from self, peer and facilitator.

Although Barrows' reiterative PBL is probably the purest form of what has been called PBL, there have been many different approaches used. Dolmans et al. (2005) indicate that "Although PBL differs in various schools, three characteristics can be considered as essential: problems as a stimulus for learning, tutors as facilitators and group work as stimulus for interaction" (p. 735). While the "McMaster Philosophy" had three key features: self-directed learning, problem-based learning, and small group tutorial learning, the only characteristic that is common among PBL forms is that learning is based upon patient problems.

PBL Problems

From a curriculum or course design perspective, you have to be clear about what you want to accomplish from PBL and plan accordingly. The focal points of curriculum planning are the PBL problems. The content of the problems needs to be carefully considered as well as the organization and timing.

There are seven qualities of an appropriate problem that have been delineated:

1. Present a common problem that graduates would be expected to be able to handle, and be prototypical of that problem.
2. Be serious or potentially serious – where appropriate management might affect the outcome.

3. Have implications for prevention.
4. Provide interdisciplinary input and cover a broad content area.
5. Lead students to address the intended objectives.
6. Present an actual (concrete) task.
7. Have a degree of complexity appropriate for the students' prior knowledge (Albanese and Mitchell 1993).

The structure or format of the problem, sometimes called a case, provides room for much variability. They can range from brief paragraphs describing a symptom or set of symptoms (e.g., chest pain) to elaborate paper or computer simulations or even using simulated patients. They can be relatively unorganized, unsynthesized, and open-ended, or they can be relatively highly structured with specific questions that need to be addressed. Barrows (1985) suggests open-ended problems, which promote application of clinical reasoning skills, structuring of knowledge in useful contexts, and development of self-directed learning. In the same curriculum, some problems can be highly structured, particularly early in the curriculum and others unstructured, especially as students approach the end of the curriculum. An example of a type of problem that is relatively structured is the Focal Problem developed at Michigan State University. It starts with a written narrative of a clinical problem as it unfolds in a real-life setting. In this design, after descriptions of significant developments occur, "stop and think" questions are inserted for students to ponder. This approach helps students focus on the steps in the decision-making process used in solving problems that may have more than one viable solution (Jones et al. 1984; Wales and Stager 1972; Pawlak et al. 1989). These varied problem designs and computer-based variants may all have a role at some point in a PBL curriculum. More structured formats might be better placed early in the curriculum when students will be challenged with even the simplest clinical scenarios while the lesser structured formats may be more effective after students gain clinical experience and comfort with the PBL method.

In curriculum design, you have to determine whether PBL will be used just for students to learn the basic sciences or whether it will continue into what are considered the clinical years. The topics and structure of the problems need to be carefully considered and tailored to the developing competency of students. The number of problems addressed needs to be considered. If problems are addressed in weeklong blocks, then the curriculum design for PBL is a sequence of problems equal to the number of weeks in the curriculum. The flow of the problems in terms of content, objectives and level of structure then becomes the backbone of the curriculum.

Student Groups

Next to the problems, the most important component of PBL is the grouping of students to work on the problem. As noted above, small groups of 6–8 are usually recommended. If the groups are too large, less assertive students have a reduced opportunity to provide input into deliberations and it gets difficult to schedule time for group meetings.

It is probably best to assign students to groups at random and to avoid including students who are couples (dating, married or otherwise related) in the same group. To the extent possible, groups should be comparable in their range of ability similar to the range for the entire class. It has become increasingly clear that just throwing a group of students together with a problem is not necessarily going to yield something useful. Guidelines and role assignments are often recommended to help students get a start in how to organize themselves to do productive work. Barrows (1985) (see pp. 60–61) recommends that students assume three separate administrative roles to make the process work smoothly: PBL reader, Action Master List Handler, and Recorder. New students should assume these roles with each new problem.

Effective groups establish basic norms of acceptable behavior. For example, the group should determine when interruption is permitted, the attitudes towards late-comers, whether eating is allowed during a session, what to do if the tasks for the day are completed early and so on. Technology is also becoming an issue for small group management and may interfere with problem-solving in any number of ways. Computers, cell phones, PDAs, MP3 players, etc., can all be used for distracting purposes. Ground rules for the use of technology should be part of the standards of acceptable behavior (e.g., no checking email, or receiving non-emergency phone calls during the session).

Small Group Facilitator

The next major participant is the facilitator(s). Who should be a facilitator has been a somewhat controversial matter. There is some evidence that having content "expert" facilitators improves student performance, especially early in the curriculum. However, it is unrealistic to have facilitators who are expert in all areas that are the subject of PBL cases. Some schools actively avoid selecting content expert facilitators to reduce student dependence upon them as information sources. Facilitators need knowledge sufficient to achieve a level of familiarity with the material. Typically facilitators need to work through a case three times to achieve what has been called "case expertness" (Zeitz and Paul 1993).

What facilitators mostly need is adequate preparation for their role. They need to be given specific guidelines for how they are to interact with students. Moving from content expert to facilitator is not necessarily a natural act for many faculty, so having them practice their role during training will be helpful. The use of "standardized" students, a group of people who are trained to act like students, can make the practice closer to the real thing. However, it can be expensive and the fidelity of the simulation to real life may be difficult to maintain.

Facilitators should also be given all information about the case and any associated readings or materials that students will be given, but in addition, materials that will allow them to be able to guide students in their search for knowledge. This includes the "next steps" that students are expected to take. If there are preparatory lectures, it will benefit the facilitators to attend. Anything that can help facilitators function in a facilitator role and achieve case expertness is useful.

Facilitators also need to be prepared for students' reaction to the experience. If students are used to having faculty serving as content deliverers, not facilitators, the transition to this type of relationship can be rocky. Facilitators need to be prepared for student frustration early in the process when the facilitator does not give them direct answers to their questions. Over time, students learn that the facilitator is explicitly not to be a source of answers to their questions, but early on it can be a difficult adjustment for students and facilitators.

How many facilitators per group (or how many groups per facilitator) is as much a practical consideration as one that is educational. The obvious answer is at least one facilitator per group would be ideal. However, faculty resources are often quite limited. A number of schools have successfully used more advanced students as facilitators or as a co-facilitator with a faculty member. There have also been studies that examined the impact of having faculty facilitate more than one group at once, circulating between them. When the facilitator cannot be with a group throughout its deliberations, it makes it difficult for the facilitator to re-engage with the group and it takes additional time that must be factored into the process. A circulating facilitator is also limited in their ability to ensure that there is balanced input from all members of the group and assess student contributions to the group process.

In summary, the qualifications of the facilitators are probably not as important as their familiarity and comfort with the cases. How many facilitators are needed depends upon how many groups and the number of facilitators used per group and the availability of facilitators. Advanced students have been used as co-facilitators with faculty to good advantage. Using fewer than one facilitator per group has significant trade-offs in terms of the facilitator's ability to manage disruptive or dysfunctional group dynamics and to evaluate student contributions to the group process.

PBL Process

The actual process used in conducting PBL can vary, but the Maastricht 7 Step method (Wood 2003) is often used as a guide for facilitators and students:

Step 1 – Identify and clarify unfamiliar terms presented in the scenario; scribe lists those that remain unexplained after discussion.

Step 2 – Define the problem or problems to be discussed; students may have different views on the issues, but all should be considered; scribe records a list of agreed problems.

Step 3 – "Brainstorming" session to discuss the problem(s), suggesting possible explanations on basis of prior knowledge; students draw on each other's knowledge and identify areas of incomplete knowledge; scribe records all discussion.

Step 4 – Review steps 2 and 3 and arrange explanations into tentative solutions; scribe organizes the explanations and restructures if necessary.

Step 5 – Formulate learning objectives; group reaches consensus on the learning objectives; tutor ensures learning objectives are focused, achievable, comprehensive, and appropriate.

Step 6 – Private study (all students gather information related to each learning objective).

Step 7 – Group shares results of private study (students identify their learning resources and share their results); tutor checks learning and may assess the group.

Grading Student Performance

Evaluating student performance in PBL is challenging. To treat it adequately would take a separate publication all by itself, perhaps a text. One of the difficulties in evaluating PBL is that the process used to solve a problem is often as important as the solution reached. Further, problem-solving in a facilitated small group is a complex task that involves social interactions and that unfolds sequentially over time. Capturing such skills in an assessment is difficult. For example, knowledge assessments have been used to assess students in PBL curricula, but they do not lend themselves very effectively for capturing the interactions that occurred during the small group sessions. Facilitator ratings would probably be better, but having facilitators rate student performance can affect group dynamics. And, if students are used as facilitators or co-facilitators, the situation becomes even more complex.

Two measures are heavily linked to PBL that are worth describing: Triple jump exercise and Objective Structured Clinical Exams (OSCEs). The primary goal of a triple jump exercise is to assess clinical problem-solving and self-directed learning skills. In a triple jump exercise, students discuss a written clinical scenario and identify the related learning goals, review the learning materials individually, and return to present their conclusions and judge their own performances. Students sometimes have 3 h to complete their exercise, sometimes a week. This type of assessment is often used for formative evaluation purposes. It is less often used for grading purposes because it is time consuming and limits the number of scenarios that can be evaluated. As a result scores tend to be contextually bound to the specific problem assessed. I personally think the name choice is unfortunate because it is too close to the negative term "jumping through hoops."

Objective Structured Clinical Examinations are performance-based examinations in which students rotate from station to station (Harden et al. 1975). At each station, students are required to do a particular task or sequence of tasks (e.g., interview a patient and perform a physical exam and then write up their assessment). There are two general types of OSCE stations, the long and short type. The long type of station can take up to a couple of hours to complete and is very extensive. The short type is much more focused and stations generally take from 10 to 15 min. The Clinical Skills portion of the United States Medical Licensure Examination Step 2 is of the short type. For the first 15 years of their existence, OSCEs were not widely adopted for high stakes evaluation purposes due to a pervasive problem with what was termed content specificity. Student performance varied quite markedly when even small changes in the nature of the content of a station were made. In the late 1980s and early 1990s, a series of studies (Colliver et al. 1989; Petrusa et al. 1991) applied generalizability theory to the problem. They were able to project acceptable reliability for OSCEs for making pass–fail decisions with at least ten stations however, reliability was found to vary dramatically between schools (Berkson 1993; Dolmans et al. 2005) and needs to be assessed with each application. OSCEs have achieved widespread adoption since that time. Stations often use standardized patients, computer simulations, literature search facilities, manikins, and other types of "hands-on" experiences. The strengths of the OSCE are its face validity and standardized clinical experience for all examinees. There are relatively few other ways of assessing complex skills and abilities such as communication skills with the same degree of standardization and reliability. The primary limitation of the OSCE pertains to the resources needed for implementation. For an in-depth discussion of the use of OSCEs in any curriculum, see Chap. 11. For readers who are interested in a thorough treatment of assessment of students in PBL, Nendaz and Tekian (1999) provide an overview. For an analysis of the strengths and weaknesses of various approaches to student assessment, see Chap. 11.

Resources

PBL can be resource intensive depending upon how it is implemented. However, a lecture-based learning curriculum is also resource intensive. It has been estimated that for class sizes less than 100, PBL may have a cost advantage (Albanese and Mitchell 1993). However, the costs of computing and the like have come down since then, but faculty time has generally become more expensive. With the rising cost of faculty time for serving as facilitators, the breakeven point between lecture and PBL has become less favorable to PBL.

In the early implementations of PBL, small groups were given dedicated space. Those who have dedicated space generally think it is very important for creating a sense of group cohesion and giving the group a place to meet at any time. It also helps to justify the tuition that many schools charge! However, dedicated space in today's crowded health sciences learning centers can be hard to come by and increasingly hard to justify. As schools respond to the anticipated shortage of physicians by increasing class sizes, they will be even more hard-pressed to supply dedicated space for PBL groups. While it is not hard to see how dedicated space would be a desirable feature, it is not necessarily clear that the lack of dedicated space will have detrimental effects on student learning.

What all small groups will need is access to information resources. Having dedicated space for groups enabled institutions to furnish them with secured computers that could be used for searching the literature or the web. However, with the increasing availability of notebook computers and remote access to the web, dedicated space for information access is not as critical. Students can even meet at the local coffee shop and have web access, something they may actually prefer. Generally, each group should have at least one computer available during their meetings. The computer is needed for recording the proceedings and accessing information resources. If a single person serves as the recorder and manages access to the information resources, some of the potential problems associated with abuse of technology can be minimized.

A well-stocked library is an important need for students in a PBL curriculum. Nolte et al. (1988) found that library use of reserve books increased 20 fold after introducing a PBL course on neurobiology into the curriculum. With the more recent advent of the internet and online references, having internet access is essential. Literature search software such as PubMed is critical. Having general web-searching capability is useful for looking for non-library references such as policy statements and current events. However, as noted by Kerfoot and colleagues (2005), there need to be guidelines for internet usage to avoid having the problem solving process subverted by web searches and non-authoritative sources.

Also beneficial are whiteboards or blackboards. Some schools have adopted electronic blackboards that enable electronic capturing of the material students write on the board. Lectures can also be an instructional resource, but Barrows recommends limiting them to 1–1.5 h per day (Barrows 1985). Barrows also recommends that basic science research faculty should be a resource available to meet with students for 4–6 h per week.

With new learners, there is a danger of having too many resource options. They can bog down looking for information and give too little attention to problem-solving. The facilitator should be quick to intervene should it happen.

The instructional environment in the small group should be informal and as low stress as possible. Lighting should be sufficient to see all the types of educational resources that will be shared. The environment (chairs) should be comfortable, but not so comfortable as to make it difficult for students to stay alert. Students should be able to bring food and drink into the meeting room. Ready access to a refrigerator and even microwave help to make the room comfortable.

Summary

Beginning a PBL curriculum is not for the faint-hearted. There is much infrastructure that needs to be put into place and there may be increased costs. While the effectiveness of PBL appears to be gaining better documentation and we are gaining a better understanding about how to do PBL, there is still much we need to learn. In the meantime, it is important to keep in mind what one is trying to accomplish with PBL. Based upon recent learning principles, Dolmans et al. (2005) identified four important processes (constructive, self-directed, collaborative and contextual) underlying PBL that provide a good synopsis of what one is trying to accomplish. By a constructive process, it is meant that learning is an active process by which students "construct or reconstruct their knowledge networks." A self-directed process is one where learners are involved in planning, monitoring and evaluating the learning process. A collaborative learning process is one in which the social structure involves two or more students interacting in which they: have a common goal, share responsibilities, are mutually dependent and need to reach agreement through open interaction. A contextual process recognizes that learning is context-bound and that transfer to different contexts requires confronting cases or problems from multiple perspectives. No matter how one decides to ultimately implement PBL, it is important that they design their experience to keep clearly in mind what they are trying to accomplish and not get distracted from their goal.

References

Albanese MA, Mitchell S (1993) Problem-based learning: a review of literature on its outcomes and implementation issues. Acad Med 68:52–81

Barrows HS (1985) How to design a problem-based curriculum for the preclinical years. Springer, New York

Barrows HS (1986) A taxonomy of problem-based learning methods. Med Educ 20:481–486

Berkson L (1993) Problem-based learning. Have the expectations been met? Acad Med 68:S79–S88

Cohen J (1988) Statistical power analysis for the behavioral sciences, 2nd edn. Lawrence Erlbaum Associates Publishers, Hillsdale

Colliver J (2000) Effectiveness of problem based learning curricula. Acad Med 75:259–266

Colliver JA, Verhulst SJ, Williams R, Norcini JJ (1989) Reliability of performance on standardized patient cases: a comparison of consistency measures based on generalizability theory. Teach Learn Med 1(1):31–37

Dolmans DHJM, De Grave W, Wolfhagen IHAP, van der Vleuten CPM (2005) Problem-based learning: future challenges for educational practice and research. Med Educ 39:732–741

Farrell T, Albanese MA, Pomrehn P (1999) Problem-based learning in ophthalmology: a pilot program for curricular renewal. Arch Ophthalmol 117:1223–1226

Harden RM, Stevenson M, Downie WW, Wilson GM (1975) Assessment of clinical competence using objective structured examination. Br Med J 1:447–451

Jones JW, Bieber LL, Echt R, Scheifley V, Ways PO (1984) A problem-based curriculum – ten years of experience. In: Schmidt HG, de Volder ML (eds) Tutorials in problem-based learning. Van Gorcum, Assen/Maastricht

Kerfoot BP, Masser BA, Hafler JP (2005) Influence of new educational technology on problem-based learning at Harvard Medical School. Med Educ 39(4):380–387

Nendaz MR, Tekian A (1999) Assessment in problem-based learning medical schools: a literature review. Teach Learn Med 11(4):232–243

Nolte J, Eller P, Ringel SP (1988) Shifting toward problem-based learning in a medical school neurobiology course. In: Research in medical education. Proceedings of the twenty-seventh annual conference. Association of American Medical Colleges, Washington, DC, pp 66–71

Pawlak SM, Popovich NG, Blank JW, Russell JD (1989) Development and validation of guided design scenarios for problem-solving instruction. Am J Pharm Educ 53:7–16

Petrusa ER, Blackwell T, Carline J, Ramsey P, McGahie W, Colindres R, Kowlowitz V, Mast T, Soler NA (1991) A multi-institutional trial of an objective structured clinical examination. Teach Learn Med 3:86–94

Vernon DTA, Blake RL (1993) Does problem-based learning work? A meta-analysis of evaluative research. Acad Med 68:550–563

Wales CE, Stager R (1972) Design of an educational system. Eng Educ 62:456–459

Wood DF (2003) ABC of learning and teaching in medicine: problem based learning. Br Med J 326:328–330

Zeitz HJ, Paul H (1993) Facilitator expertise and problem-based learning in PBL and traditional curricula. Acad Med 68(3):203–204

Chapter 6
Team-Based Learning

Dean X. Parmelee and Azzam S. Al-Kadi

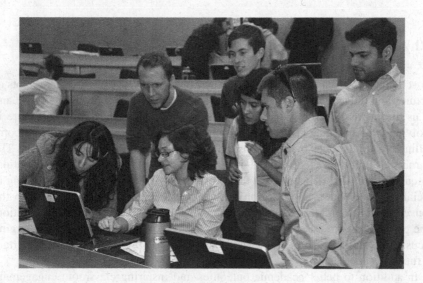

Abstract Team-Based Learning (TBL) is a large group, peer teaching method that can also be described as an expert-led, interactive and analytical teaching strategy. TBL keeps the class together (large group) with one or more expert(s) while the students apply the content to specific problems (analytical) in small groups (interactive) at intervals during the learning session. The students are expected to prepare prior to the session. Content is *used* throughout the session rather than simply introduced. This approach allows students to practice with the content under the watchful eye of the expert.

D.X. Parmelee, M.D., FAACAP., FAPA (✉)
Boonschoft School of Medicine, Wright State University,
3640 Colonel Glenn Hwy, Dayton, OH 45435, USA
e-mail: dean.parmelee@wright.edu

A.S. Al-Kadi, M.D., M.Sc., FRCSC
Unaizah College of Medicine, Qassim University, Qassim, Saudi Arabia

K.N. Huggett and W.B. Jeffries (eds.), *An Introduction to Medical Teaching*,
DOI 10.1007/978-94-017-9066-6_6, © Springer Science+Business Media Dordrecht 2014

Introduction

Team-Based Learning (TBL) is an instructional strategy that uses the power of small group learning within the large classroom setting. It works well with class sizes as small as a dozen to as large as over 200, depending on space design and acoustics. For the learner, it requires considerable accountability to come on time, come prepared, and engage collaboratively with a small group of peers to solve problems and make decisions. For the instructor, it requires subject matter expertise, adherence to the structure and process of the strategy, and the conviction that the best use of one's time in the classroom is to uncover content, not cover it. Done correctly, it transforms the learning culture. TBL enables learners to become more self-directed, but also fosters their ability to work with others. For the instructor, TBL augments the vitality of the experience by applying expertise at the point of learning.

Why Do TBL?

Most faculty have learned to teach from their own experiences as a student – lots of lectures and didactic sessions to cover content for a test. What would motivate any of us to do this differently, since we all turned out just fine? Although there is evolving evidence that TBL leads to improved academic outcomes, a more compelling reason emerges by either observing or participating in a TBL session. The learners are fully engaged with the material and each other, analyzing information, speculating, making decisions that they can defend. No one is napping, engaging in social media or other activities on their computer. The instructor listens to the conversations around the room and when teams display their choices to a question, s/he probes some of the teams to explain their reasoning processes. The emerging focus of the session becomes the "why" and "how" to a problem, which is important to future practice.

In addition to better academic outcomes and inspiring classroom engagement with the learners, another important reason for using TBL is that instructors often discover they prefer this modality to passive large group teaching methods. TBL focuses on application of knowledge and building of skill. For example, if you teach something about acid-base balance, can your presentation ever reassure you that the students both understand it and apply this knowledge to the solution of a clinical problem? No, of course not – they will only truly grasp the principles through solving progressively challenging problems – with you there to coach, probe, and affirm them when they achieve the desired objectives.

In practice, TBL teaches students how to solve any problem while being part of a team, similar to real practice where health professionals from different disciplines work together to manage medical problems. In TBL, team spirit and collaboration between team members develops early. With the increasing focus on patient safety in health care settings, TBL provides students with many opportunities to learn how to better communicate and collaborate in the team setting.

How Did TBL Develop?

In the early 1990s, a business school professor, Dr. Larry Michaelsen, became frustrated with lecturing to increasingly large classes. He could never tell whether his students were paying attention or if they could apply what they were hearing. Furthermore, he wanted his students to leave his classes and be able to use what they learned when they went into business for themselves. He wanted to give them examples of "real life" problems they would face and ensure they knew how to make the best decisions. He thus designed a novel instructional strategy that used the power of small groups (teams) to solve authentic problems through consensus-building discussions and to defend them in the whole class setting. Students learned quickly to come to class fully-prepared as individuals – there was a "test" at the beginning, followed by the same test taken as a team. An individual student's grade in the course depended upon his/her individual effort AND how the team performed. To promote student accountability to the group, a peer evaluation component was introduced to the grading.

Dr. Michaelsen's strategy became very popular with his students, other faculty started to use it, and students started asking for its use in more classes. Since its introduction, there have been many peer-reviewed publications in the higher education literature on the effectiveness of TBL. In 2001, Dr. Boyd Richards at the Baylor College of Medicine received a grant from the U.S. Department of Education to help health professions institutions explore and use TBL. This grant inspired many U.S. medical, dental, nursing, and allied health schools to learn more and implement TBL. This has resulted in many publications by health professions educators on effectiveness, strategies for implementation, and clarification and refinement of the method (Koles et al. 2010; Haidet et al. 2012; Thomas and Bowen 2011; Parmelee et al. 2012; Levine et al. 2004). The grant established the *Team-Based Learning Collaborative (TLBC)*, an international organization of educators from secondary through post-graduate programs in higher education. Through its dynamic website, annual meetings, regional workshops, practitioner database, and listserv, a learning community has evolved along with scholarship of teaching and learning on the strategy (http://www.teambasedlearning.org).

What Are the Components of TBL?

To implement TBL, five essential components must be considered.

- Advanced Preparation – Students need to know what they must learn before coming to class and at what level of mastery. Preparation may include readings, attending lectures, completing dissection, patient examination or laboratory assignments. To encourage their lifelong learning skills, clarify that your Advanced Preparation assignment is the minimum for preparation, and that they can identify their own and additional learning objectives for the unit of study. Over time, students will do this, not so much for any grade enhancement, but to contribute more to their team discussions!

- Readiness Assurance – first an individually-administered multiple choice question (MCQ) test is administered based on material taken directly from the Advanced Preparation (Individual Readiness Assurance Test – iRAT) followed by a Team Readiness Assurance Test (tRAT), using an Immediate Feedback Assessment Technique (IF-AT, see below). Discussion of difficult questions is directed by the instructor to assure clarification of key facts and concepts in preparation for the Group Application. As throughout TBL, the instructor does not provide a lecture here, just Socratic-style dialogue with teams on their decisions, getting teams to teach other teams. An Appeals process should be available to address points of ambiguity, but should not slow the class down.
- Group Application – this is a question or a set of questions the answers for which cannot be found in the books or on the internet but only through in-depth discussion within teams. There are data to analyze, interpret or synthesize with other information. A specific choice must be made by each team, either in a MCQ format or another format that makes it easy for display for full class discussion. The problems posed in the Group Application are just like the ones to be solved in real life as a practitioner. By design, this is the most important part of a TBL module – the one where students should feel that they are learning how to apply what they have learned about the subject.
- Instructor Summary – the instructor seizes the opportunity to reflect on what has been learned and accomplished in the module, clarifies any remaining misunderstandings, and asks students what else they feel they need to learn or do to become "expert."
- Peer Feedback and Evaluation – this is done about halfway through a course for practice, then at the end for a grade. There are a variety of formats, but all ask students to provide honest and forthright feedback to teammates about what each has contributed to each others learning and how they might contribute more in the future.

What Do Students Experience with TBL?

As indicated above, students become very engaged with learning both outside and inside the classroom. As one can imagine, it can be unpopular to tell students that the next time they come to class they will have a test on new content that they must learn on their own. Thus students should be carefully introduced to the structure of TBL. How does this happen? The instructor can demonstrate how TBL works by doing a practice module:

- Give learners 15 min to read an article/paper
- Administer a five question test (MCQ format) about the material
- Administer a team test in which small groups of 5–7 students take the same test together

- Use the Immediate Feedback Assessment Technique (IF-AT, http://www. epsteineducation.com/home/about/) to achieve consensus decisions on the questions
- Ask students "What has just happened?" with their learning
- Give students a question that requires them to work in the same teams and apply what they learned so far
- Conclude with dialogue on this brief experience and outline how the next one will be conducted

What Does the Instructor Need to Do to Get Started with TBL?

First, one should consider the appropriate educational design for TBL. Whether one is developing a single TBL module to "field test" or designing an entire course that will include TBL as an instructional strategy, the place to start is with good "Backward Design" (Wiggins and McTighe 1998). At its simplest, this means doing these three things:

- Define what you want your learners to be able to do with what they learn by the end of a unit of study. Bloom et al. (1956) defined progressively more challenging expectations of learning that begin with knowledge, progress to understanding, application, analysis, synthesis and evaluation. In TBL, do not settle for what you want them to know or understand. Make the leap to higher levels of learning, such as application, analysis, and synthesis. Being clear about this empowers you to write your goals and objectives with a language that is outcome-based and measurable. Consider this example from Human Anatomy and ask which learning objective is better for your students' future careers?

  - List and describe the muscles, tendons, fascia and skeletal features of the brachial plexus.
  - Given a case description of a patient with a shoulder injury, be able to analyze the problem by localizing the injury level and its extent, characterize its impact on limb/body function, and design -with justification- a multimodality approach to manage patient's injury

- Determine how to assess whether your learners have accomplished your goals and objectives at the end of the unit. Identify the evidence that will assure you and them that they understand and can apply what they have learned.
- Design the teaching and learning activities that will provide the students with the greatest opportunities to accomplish the unit's goals and objectives. This should include in-class and out-of-class activities. Keeping the brachial plexus example in mind, consider a combination of activities such as: a lecture (live or online) using images (moving and static) of the anatomical structures and relationships; guided dissection of the area or programmed study of a prosection; in-class or online case problems that give practice in how to diagnose an injury to the region; a TBL module where the Group Application is case-focused and builds on knowing the detailed anatomy from the dissection.

The second step is to design and write the Group Application for one TBL module. To do this well, you must adhere to the 4 S's (Michaelsen and Sweet 2007):

- Significant Problem – Choose a problem, situation, or case that is both authentic and representative of the kind of problem the students will encounter in their professional careers. In medical education there is no shortage of good case material, and when presented well, the students know that you are selecting a meaningful problem.
- Specific Choice – Structure the question or questions so that they must make a specific choice. Remember, decision-making is close to the heart of TBL, and nothing generates as much passion within a group (or angst in an individual) than having to decide among similar options. Sometimes, all of the options you pose are good, but given the particular context of the problem and how one interprets the data, one can endorse a BEST option. WARNING – this is the greatest challenge for the instructor – anticipating how students will process a set of data and formulating plausible choice options.
- Same Problem – By having all teams working on the same problem at the same time, you avoid one of the greatest pitfalls of large class/small group activities. Most students will have had the experience of working with a small group of students in or out of a class, each group working on a different but related topic, and being required to present the findings to the whole class. This is a colossal waste of time: students who are not presenting their findings are not paying attention; once a group has presented, they feel done and tune out; the individual student may learn something about their group's assignment, but very little about the others. In TBL, everyone stays engaged because they want to defend their team's choice and, in so doing, they learn when questioned by other teams.
- Simultaneous Reporting – In TBL, all teams display their choices at the same time. Why? This does two things: every team invests in their choice since it has to be seen by all, no escape; every team gets feedback on their choice in comparison to all the other teams – they know where they stand. The instructor strategizes on the spot how to generate the most debate on the choices displayed, which should be the golden teaching opportunity of the module.

The third step is to prepare the Readiness Assurance Test. This should use the MCQ format, and the quality and difficulty level of the questions should be equivalent to the course's final exam. Students appreciate well-constructed Readiness Assurance Tests because they provide feedback on how well they are learning the content and they should predict how they will perform on any summative exams.

Step Four is to select the best resources for the students to learn the content. Besides textbooks, articles, and lecture material, one can include problem sets, fieldwork, patient interviews, reflective essays, anything that you feel facilitates preparation for the Group Application and the Readiness Assurance. If in the course of the whole class discussion, a team makes an important point or observation that has evolved from their going deeper into the content with other sources, be sure to highlight this for the class. Students often go beyond the minimum and establish additional learning objectives for concepts or topics they feel will be important.

What Are the Greatest Obstacles to Success with TBL?

There are several things that can go wrong with implementing TBL into a course or curriculum – here are some of them:

- Course planning: If the TBL module or modules do not link meaningfully with the rest of the content, then the students will not feel that the time they spend in TBL is worth it. TBLs have to be tightly integrated with the content and not perceived as appendages.
- Module design: It takes considerable time and effort to construct a good TBL module. Creating one is much more difficult than putting together a few lectures. It also has a better chance of success if it is peer reviewed by colleagues and students. Allow plenty of time for this, but remember that once you have a good one, you can use it again and again.
- Little details: Make sure your materials for a module are well prepared, proofread, and organized. There will not be time in a live session to make corrections to materials or fix a major clerical or administrative error, e.g., the IF-AT form is not coded correctly for the question set.
- Facilitation: Take some time to attend a faculty development workshop on TBL and learn how to facilitate a module. There are lots of little tricks you can add to enhance the classroom experience for your students and yourself. For example, use the PICKME! App (http://www.classeapps.com/pick-me) to select students at random to respond to your questions rather than ask for a volunteer; require students to stand when they speak and address to the whole class; "listen in" to as many team discussions as you can during the periods when they are making decisions and use what you learn about how they are thinking to probe further in the class discussion phase; and never exceed 2 ½ h in any one session because the students will drift off from fatigue. You can always split up a module, e.g., do the Readiness Assurance in one time period and the Group Application in another. Always allow a few minutes at the end BEFORE they start packing their bags to summarize what you feel they have learned and ask for feedback on the day.
- Facilities: There are ideal classrooms for TBL, but usually you won't have them. The quality of your materials and your facilitation skills either make or break a module. However, it does help if you have space in which your team numbers are visible from throughout the room and the students can cluster easily. Rooms with large round tables are the least conducive to TBL. The students will have a hard time clustering and they'll move to spaces between the tables. If you are invited by your administration to help plan the next education building, contact some of the consultants on the TBLC website for input.

Summary

TBL is a well thought-out and proven instructional strategy that is being used increasingly in medical education around the globe. It has several components that address the professional competencies of the health care professional: self-directed learning, teamwork, interpersonal communication, peer instruction and feedback. There is significant evidence for the academic outcomes of TBL (i.e., summative exam performance). Students prefer TBL over other types of small group learning, and much prefer it to hours of passive lectures. Because it has a defined structure that works, novice instructors are advised to follow the process carefully to have the greatest chance of success. There are many good resources in the literature and TBL websites for one to learn more about how to implement TBL and connect with practitioners from several disciplines within medicine.

References

Engelhart MD, Furst EJ, Hill WH, Krathwohl DR (1956) Taxonomy of educational objectives: the classification of educational goals. In: Bloom BS (ed) Handbook 1: cognitive domain. David McKay, New York

Haidet P, Levine RE, Parmelee DX, Crow S, Kennedy F, Kelly PA, Perkowski L, Michaelsen LK, Richards BF (2012) Perspective: guidelines for reporting team-based learning activities in the medical and health sciences education literature. Acad Med 87(3):292–299

Koles PG, Stolfi A, Borges NJ, Nelson S, Parmelee DX (2010) The impact of team-based learning on medical students' academic performance. Acad Med 85:1739–1745

Levine RE, Haidet P, Lynn DJ, Stone JJ, Wolf DV, Paniagua FA (2004) Transforming a clinical clerkship with team learning. Teach Learn Med 16(3):270–275

Michaelsen LK, Sweet M (2007) Creating effective team assignments. In: Michaelsen LK, Parmelee DX, McMahon KK, Levine RE (eds) Team-based learning for health professions education: a guide to using small groups for improving learning. Stylus Publishing, Sterling

Parmelee DX, Michaelsen L, Cook S, Hudes P (2012) Team-based learning: a practical guide, AMEE guide no. 65. Dundee: AMEE, 34(5)

Thomas PA, Bowen CW (2011) A controlled trial of team-based learning in an ambulatory medicine clerkship for medical students. Teach Learn Med 23:31–36

Wiggins G, McTighe JH (1998) Understanding by design. Merrill Prentice Hall, Columbus

Chapter 7
Teaching Clinical Skills

Janet M. Riddle

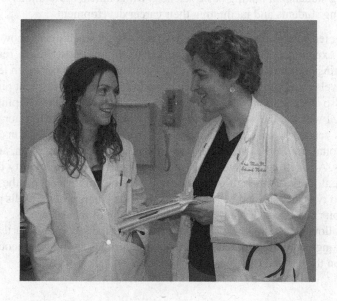

Abstract Being a clinician teacher is exciting and stimulating. Most clinician teachers simply enjoy teaching and value contributing to the development of young professionals. Clinicians also find that teaching keeps their knowledge and skills up to date. Clinical teachers are asked to fulfill a variety of roles. This chapter focuses on specific and effective strategies for enhancing student learning in the clinical setting through inquiry and effective feedback.

J.M. Riddle, M.D. (✉)
Department of Medical Education, University of Illinois-Chicago College
of Medicine, Chicago, IL, USA
e-mail: jriddle@uic.edu

K.N. Huggett and W.B. Jeffries (eds.), *An Introduction to Medical Teaching*,
DOI 10.1007/978-94-017-9066-6_7, © Springer Science+Business Media Dordrecht 2014

Introduction

Being a clinician teacher is exciting and stimulating. Most clinician teachers simply enjoy teaching and value contributing to the development of young professionals. Clinicians also find that teaching keeps their knowledge and skills up to date. Clinical teachers are asked to fulfill a variety of roles. These include:

- Serving as a physician role model – exemplifying competent professional care of patients
- Teaching and reinforcing clinical skills
- Being a supervisor – providing opportunities for students to practice clinical skills with patients
- Observing and providing feedback on student performance
- Assisting students in linking basic sciences with clinical correlations
- Mentoring students and facilitating their career development

Learning teaching skills, including how to prepare for teaching and how to reflect on clinical experiences, will increase your satisfaction with teaching. Teaching in clinical settings is characterized by diversity. You may be asked to teach learners at different levels of training – from first-year medical students to resident physicians. You may also teach pharmacy students, nursing students or a multidisciplinary team of learners. I will use the word "student" throughout this chapter to refer to any of the learners you teach. Clinical teaching occurs in a variety of settings – in outpatient clinics, hospital wards, the emergency department, in the operating room, and during home visits. Any setting in which you care for patients is an opportunity for you to teach clinical skills. Although your teaching will be influenced by the kinds of patients you typically see and by the level of students you teach, the skills presented in this chapter can be used in any setting and with any of these learners.

In the following sections, we will explore each of the key phases of teaching in clinical settings: planning for teaching, teaching during the clinical encounter, and reflecting on the clinical experience (Irby 1992).

Planning for Teaching Clinical Skills

As you plan for clinical teaching, you need to understand the goals and objectives that the course or clerkship director has for the clinical experience in which you are teaching. What are students expected to know or to be able to do as a result of your teaching? It will help you to know how the course or clerkship that you are teaching in relates to other courses and clinical experiences in the curriculum. Clinical experiences early in medical training allow students to correlate the basic sciences they are learning in the classroom with clinical problems. Later in training, students need patient care experiences to refine clinical skills and develop their fund of knowledge. You will want to plan learning activities that assist students in integrating content among courses, build on previous clinical experiences, and enhance the student's clinical capabilities.

When planning for clinical teaching, you need to consider the level of training of the student you will be working with and that student's interests and learning needs. Students early in their training are learning basic skills in interviewing and examining patients. They need opportunities both to observe you demonstrating these skills as well as opportunities to practice them with patients. Junior students are also socializing to the role of being a physician. You will want to explicitly role model professional behaviors. Students welcome mentoring that focuses on their development as novice clinicians. More advanced students are eager to refine their physical diagnosis skills. They are also developing clinical reasoning skills and capabilities in negotiating management plans with patients. Senior students are often exploring career options and are eager for your advice. Even within these generalizations, there are individual differences. You should plan to discuss goals and learning needs with each student.

Orienting Students to Facilitate Clinical Teaching

Orienting the student to your clinical setting is an important step in planning for clinical teaching (Alguire et al. 2008). An orientation eases the student's transition to working with you and your patients. During the orientation, be sure to explain your routines in patient care. Also introduce the student to anyone else you work with, for instance nursing staff, office staff or pharmacists. Consider what the student might learn from each of these people. Medical assistants can teach students to measure blood pressure or blood sugar. Pharmacists can teach students about medication counseling. Students value diverse experiences in clinical settings and appreciate the importance of learning to work on a healthcare team.

During the orientation, describe to the student how you provide clinical supervision and teaching. This is a key step in establishing a positive learning climate. Students value clinical teachers who are enthusiastic about teaching, who inspire confidence in students' knowledge and skills, who provide feedback, and who encourage students to accept responsibility for patient care. Being enthusiastic about teaching is demonstrated by asking students about themselves and their learning needs. Students appreciate your efforts to provide them with clinical experiences that are relevant to their learning needs and their stage of development. Describe for the student how clinical encounters will occur. Should the student expect to "shadow" you for some encounters? How will you observe the student's clinical skills? What information do you want included in case presentations? What kinds of notes do you expect the student to write? What teaching methods do you plan to use? Will you give assignments to the student? When and how will the student's final evaluation take place?

Don't forget to find out what the student expects to learn by working with you. Some clinical teachers use "learning contracts" to negotiate goals and expectations with the student (Alguire et al. 2008). These contracts can include self-assessments of clinical skills, a statement of the student's goals for the experience, and planned

Table 7.1 Keys for an effective student orientation (Alguire et al. 2008)

Review the learning goals and expectations for the clinical experience
Orient the student to your clinical site, patient care routines, and staff
Discuss your student's expectations for the experience
Explain your expectations of the student
Describe how you provide clinical supervision and teaching, including how feedback and evaluation
will occur

strategies for meeting those goals. While exploring the student's expectations, you can confirm that the student understands the goals and objectives for the experience, and that you understand the other courses and clinical experiences that the student has had. Discussing the student's career interests is also helpful (Table 7.1).

Selecting Patients for Clinical Teaching

You need to plan for each of the student's clinical encounters. Although teachable moments occur with every patient, you want to have a clear purpose for each clinical encounter that the student has. What will the student learn by working with this patient? Patients who have typical presentations of common diseases or prototypical clinical findings are good choices for students. Some clinical teachers select a general problem or theme for each session with a student. Students are able to observe a spectrum of patients with a similar diagnosis. Alternatively, by focusing on a clinical problem, students are able to compare and contrast different diagnoses with similar presentations. This assists students in developing concepts of the key features of diagnoses.

Plan to cover enough material with each patient encounter to stimulate the student's clinical thinking, but without overwhelming the student. Have one or two important teaching points for each encounter. The teaching points that you have selected should help the student meet the learning objectives for the clinical experience. Make sure that you have selected patients of manageable complexity for the student. At the beginning of each session, review the list of patients you are scheduled to see. Together you can select patients and discuss the teaching points that you have in mind.

Select patients who have good communication skills and who are willing to work with students. Many patients appreciate the extra attention that students give them. Patients understand the importance of teaching students. They know that they are contributing to the development of the next generation of physicians. Be sure to brief each patient about the "teaching encounter". Introduce the student, explain how the encounter will occur, solicit the patient's consent, and inform the patient that you will return after the student has finished the encounter. Respect your patient's decision to not to work with your student. Many clinical teachers find that modeling the kind of relationship that they would like students to have with patients is beneficial. A useful rule of thumb is to treat your students as you would like them to treat your patients.

Teaching During the Clinical Encounter

As a clinical teacher you will be best served by having a variety of teaching methods to use in different situations and with different learners. Effective clinical teachers engage students through multiple strategies (Hatem et al. 2011; Fromme et al. 2010; Sutkin et al. 2008):

- Asking questions, listening carefully, and responding effectively
- Involving students in meaningful ways – through demonstration, observation, and feedback
- Role-modeling and reflection

What is most important is that you allow students to practice skills and work with problems that will help them gain clinical competence. Let the students practice what you want them to be able to do!

Using Questions and Feedback to Enhance Clinical Reasoning

Questions play a key role in any clinical teaching. Questions stimulate and engage students; help you to determine your student's knowledge level and learning needs; and help you monitor how your students are progressing. The questions you ask can promote higher-order thinking and encourage reflection. The questions you have asked, and the student's responses, are also the basis for giving constructive feedback.

When discussing clinical cases, your questions can have three purposes – to obtain factual information, to explore the student's reasoning processes, or to explore the student's learning needs (Connell et al. 1999). A common problem with case discussions is that questions are limited to obtaining factual information. These lower-order questions ask for more information about the patient or about what the student knows. Students may also be asked to repeat or recall what they have learned. Lower-order questions may help the clinician to care for the patient, but these questions do not help students develop clinical judgment or problem-solving skills. In contrast, you can ask questions that explore the student's understanding of the patient's clinical problem – by asking the student to formulate the problem or to think through the problem (Bowen 2006). You can also probe the uncertainties or difficulties that the student is having; thereby eliciting the student's learning needs. Exploring clinical thinking and learning needs require higher-order questions – questions that ask students to summarize, analyze, compare and contrast, and justify. Higher-order questions also tend to be open-ended, thus have a range of possible responses (Table 7.2).

Table 7.2 Keys to asking effective questions

Ask one question at a time
If you ask more than one question, you increase the complexity of the learning task
Wait three seconds before and after the student answers
Give students time to organize their thoughts
Stay neutral until after the student has explained the answer
Avoid the "rapid reward" that terminates thinking
Use higher-order, open-ended questions
Create a safe environment that permits students to answer incorrectly or to guess

The METRC Model for Case-Based Teaching

I will present two models of case-based teaching. The first is the "METRC" model, a variation of the "one-minute preceptor" or "microskills" model for teaching during clinical encounters (Neher et al. 1992). The steps of the "METRC" model are:

- Make a commitment
- Explore or explain reasoning
- Teach to the gaps
- Reinforce what was done well
- Correct mistakes

After presenting a patient case to you, the student may pause or ask a question. This is your cue to ask the student to make a commitment to what she is thinking at this point. Your question allows the student to process information collected during the encounter. You are asking the student to formulate the clinical problem and to demonstrate her knowledge related to that clinical problem. Depending upon the specifics of the clinical case, your question might be "What do you think is going on with this patient?", "What is the most likely diagnosis?", "What tests would be most useful?", or "What treatment plan would you propose?" You may be tempted to ask for more factual information about the patient, but wait.

Once the student has committed to a specific diagnosis (or diagnostic strategy or treatment plan), your next question is to ask the student to explain her answer. You might ask, "What information in the history and physical led you to that diagnosis?", "What do you expect to find from the tests that you propose?", "Why did you select that medication for treating the patient, given the options available?" These questions ask students to analyze information and to justify their decisions. Two questions that are helpful to probe the student's thinking are to ask "What if the patient had …? How would that change your thinking?" and "How are … and … similar or different?" (Bowen 2006). Questions that explore the student's reasoning provide opportunities for the student to reveal additional information obtained from the patient that was omitted from the original case presentation. If you still have not heard important factual information, now is the time to ask.

After hearing the student responses to the first two steps, you know where the student's gaps in knowledge or misconceptions are. The third step in the METRC model is to teach to the gaps. In general you should teach one or two important points – but not everything that you know about the patient or the diagnosis. Your teaching should match the learning needs of the student and should develop the student's knowledge and skills. The first three steps in the METRC model may be used for a brief teaching encounter or may be repeated during a more in-depth case discussion. Your student may raise questions, which you may want to assign to the student for self-directed learning.

Each clinical encounter is an opportunity to give formative feedback to the student. The final two steps in the METRC model prompt you to do so. Begin by reinforcing what the student did well. You should describe clearly the specific desirable behaviors you observed. Then correct any mistakes you observed or make suggestions for improvement. Again, you will need to be clear and specific. I will discuss feedback in more detail later in this chapter. The important point here is that you are able to give feedback based upon the student's knowledge and skills that you have probed through the questions that you have asked.

Teaching the Student to "Prime the Preceptor"

The second model for case-based teaching, SNAPPS, is an alternative to the METRC model. In this model, the student guides the clinical teaching encounter. In SNAPPS, the student primes the clinical teacher with what he needs to know or learn from the preceptor (Wolpaw et al. 2003). The student uses the following steps in clinical case presentations:

- Summarize briefly the patient's history and physical
- Narrow the differential diagnosis to two or three most relevant possibilities
- Analyze the differential diagnosis by comparing and contrasting the diagnoses
- Probe the clinical teacher by asking questions about areas of confusion, uncertainty or knowledge deficits
- Plan management of the patient's medical issues
- Select a focused, patient-related question for self-directed learning

Students need to be taught this approach to case presentations. SNAPPS is a learner-centered model that focuses on both exploring the student's clinical reasoning and learning needs.

Teaching in the Patient's Presence

Teaching in the patient's presence involves a learning triad – the patient, the student, and you, the clinical teacher. Your task is to diagnose the patient's clinical problem along with the learner's abilities and needs. As discussed earlier in this chapter, it is important to prepare patients for their role in clinical teaching. Maintaining good communication with patients during teaching encounters involves obtaining their consent, ensuring their understanding of the discussion, and allowing them to ask questions and give feedback to both you and the student. When discussing clinical information in the patient's presence, be sure to use language that the patient can understand.

As with any clinical teaching, you should have a focused purpose for teaching in the patient's presence. Using the technique of "priming" can help the student (Alguire et al. 2008). Although priming can be used with any clinical encounter, it is especially helpful when you want to limit the time that the student spends with the patient. Simply, you identify the tasks that the student is expected to complete while with the patient and the time frame for completing the tasks. You will also want to explain what the student will have accomplished as a result of the encounter, for instance a problem-focused note or an oral presentation.

Teaching Through "Active Observation"

Demonstration plays an important part in clinical teaching. In demonstrations, you ask the student to "Watch me take care of this patient". Rather than simply having students passively observe your interactions with patients, use the technique of "active observation" (Wilkerson and Sarkin 1998). In this teaching method, begin by identifying what the student should learn from observing your interaction with a patient. You can use active observation with more junior students to role model communication skills, clinical skills – including interviewing and physical examination, and professionalism. This method can also be used in complex or difficult situations, in which the student may not have the necessary knowledge or skills. Demonstrating communication skills in giving bad news to patients is an example. After identifying the learning objective, tell the student what she should do during the encounter – What should the student pay attention to? Be sure to prepare the student for whether you will ask questions or have the student repeat parts of the physical examination. After the clinical encounter, discuss what the student observed and learned from watching you.

As an example, you have a patient who is being prepared for hospital discharge. You would like your student to observe how you counsel your patient about the medications she is being discharged on. You ask your student to pay attention to how you ask your patient to repeat the instructions you have given to make sure that she understands. After asking for the student's observations, you might continue the discussion with, "How else could we have confirmed that the patient understood the discharge instructions?"

The "Two-Minute Observation"

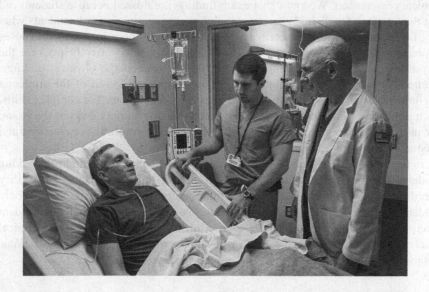

In addition to the opportunities for role modeling, teaching in the patient's presence allows you to observe your student's clinical skills. Students are rarely observed actually interacting with patients and families. Valuable opportunities for feedback are thus missed. Observations need not be detailed or time consuming. In fact it is probably better to make multiple short observations of your student. In the "two-minute observation" the clinical teacher observes the student interacting with the patient for 2 min (Wilkerson and Sarkin 1998). The teacher and student begin by establishing the objective for the observation. You may choose to focus on how the student begins the patient interview and whether the student uses open-ended questions to explore the patient's concerns. Or you may focus on how the student counsels the patient on medications or lifestyle modification. Not matter what your objective is, you will need to explain to the patient that you are observing the student and that you will return. You then make your observations and leave without disturbing the student-patient interaction. The student is now able to complete the patient visit. After the clinical encounter has concluded, give your student feedback on your observations.

Special Considerations for Teaching Physical Examination Skills

Students must perform four steps in order to make a correct diagnosis on the basis of the physical examination. Students need to anticipate the physical exam findings, perform the maneuvers necessary to elicit the findings, describe the findings that are present, and interpret the findings (Yudkowsky et al. 2009). In the first step, the student needs to anticipate what physical exam findings to look for based upon the patient's clinical presentation. We know that exam findings are missed because students did not think to look for them. When teaching physical examination, ask students what key findings they would expect based on the two or three most likely diagnoses explaining the patient's symptoms. The second step is to correctly perform the physical examination maneuvers that are needed to elicit the physical findings. Demonstration of correct techniques, followed by observation of the student's performance with feedback, are important teaching techniques. For complex skills, such as hearing heart murmurs, you may need to focus on only parts of the exam, for instance, "Listen in this area. Pay attention to what you hear between first and second heart sounds".

In the third step, the student must be able to describe the exam findings. Asking students to draw a picture of what they observed or to tap out a rhythm of what they heard can be helpful techniques to elicit their description of findings. You can help students learn the technical terms used to describe exam findings. Finally the student interprets the exam findings in the context of the patient's history. As a clinical teacher, you should emphasize each of these four steps through asking questions, demonstrating correct techniques, and providing feedback.

Special Considerations for Teaching Procedural Skills

We use a four-step approach to teaching procedures. This approach can be used to teach relatively simple procedures such as peripheral intravenous catheter insertion, phlebotomy, or obtaining an electrocardiogram. These steps can also be used to teach other "procedures" such as physical examination skills. This approach allows students to learn both the cognitive and psychomotor steps in performing a procedure. Even with this approach, a student may not be able to completely master a procedure if there are not sufficient opportunities for practice and feedback.

Involving the patient in teaching procedures is crucial. You must explain the student's role and your role in performing the procedure. It is your responsibility to obtain informed consent from the patient. You need to explain to the patient what is occurring while teaching or supervising the procedure.

In the first step, break down the procedure into its component parts (Peyton 1998). This includes more than the individual steps in correctly performing the procedure. It also includes the indications and contraindications for the procedure, as well as proper preparation and positioning of the patient, and use of the equipment. Demonstrate the procedure to the student in the second step. Perform your demonstration slowly – talking through each step. In the third step, you will perform the procedure, but the student will talk through each part of the procedure. These two steps allow the student to internalize the correct steps – without having to perform the motor skills necessary to complete the procedure.

The final step has the student actually perform the procedure, talking through each step that he is taking. This allows the student to add the motor skill component to the cognitive component. Depending upon the complexity of the procedure, it is clear that some procedures are best taught and learned on models or simulators. A clinical skills lab allows practice, repetition and feedback in a high-fidelity, low risk environment.

The "Final" Step in Clinical Teaching – Giving Constructive Feedback

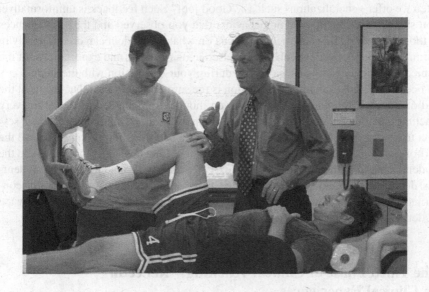

Feedback is crucial to learning. Feedback allows students to learn about their current levels of competence and allows them to reflect on their strengths and weaknesses. Through feedback, students engage in a dialogue with a clinical teacher in order to become more competent. Feedback is the information that is given to the student that is intended to guide that student's performance. Feedback should be given regularly. As suggested by the METRC model, there are opportunities for feedback in every teaching encounter.

Constructive feedback is timely, direct and clear (Sachdeva 1996; Hewson and Little 1998). Don't wait until too long after an event to give feedback. Your student will be more likely to accept your feedback and make changes, if you give feedback in a timely fashion. Be sensitive to the setting. Public areas are not conducive to well-received feedback – even if nothing "negative" is said. Students are not always aware that you are giving feedback, so start by saying, "Let me give you some feedback". Establish a positive tone. Asking your student how the rotation is going

Table 7.3 Keys to giving constructive feedback (Hewson and Little 1998)

Make sure that feedback is well-timed and expected
Ask for the student's assessment of her performance
Deal with specific behaviors that you have observed
Don't give too much feedback at one time. Instead, give feedback regularly
Offer specific suggestions for improvement. Limit feedback to remediable behaviors

is a good way to decrease some of the student's anxiety. Then ask the student to assess her performance by describing her perceptions of strengths and areas for improvement.

Feedback should deal with specific performances that you have observed. Too often we offer generalizations such as, "Good job!" Such feedback is uninformative. You should describe the specific behaviors that you observed and the consequences of those behaviors. Be constructive – focus on what the student can do differently in a similar situation. Feedback should be based upon the goals and expectations for the clinical experience that you established during your orientation with the student.

Feedback is not evaluation. Evaluation is the summative process that occurs at the end of a course, rotation or clerkship. Even though you included feedback in every teaching encounter, you should also plan for a mid-rotation summative feedback session to review the student's overall performance. You may find it helpful to use the end-of-rotation evaluation form during this session. Plan to discuss to what extent the student is meeting the objectives of the experience, what competencies the students has demonstrated, and which skills need more work. Students are typically concerned about the final evaluation or grade. In these sessions, you can discuss how the student is progressing and set goals for the remainder of the rotation (Table 7.3).

The Third Phase of Clinical Teaching – Reflecting on Clinical Experiences

Reflection is important in the learning process. Reflection on clinical experiences allows students to formulate and refine clinical concepts. The process of reflection creates additional opportunities for constructive feedback. Through reflection, students plan for and anticipate what they will do in future clinical encounters. Thus reflection prepares students for future learning.

Two specific strategies for reflection include "wrap-up rounds" and homework. During wrap-up rounds, the clinical teacher and student review the patients seen during the session. Ask the student to summarize the two or three most important points from the session. A useful question is to ask, "What did you learn today that was new for you?" Other tasks that require the student to synthesize knowledge are making charts or diagrams that explain what the student understands about the pathophysiology of the patient's clinical problem or outline the student's approach to evaluating that problem. Ask your student how he would explain the concepts learned during the session to his peers. It is also useful to ask the student to make connections between clinical experiences and classroom learning. Ask, "What are you learning in your classes that related to patients you saw today?"

Giving homework assignments is another useful reflection exercise. Reading assignments encourage self-directed, independent learning. Have your students write down the questions that they have about patients on paper or in a smartphone. Encourage them to make the question as specific as possible. The student should select one question that she decides is most important to taking care of the patient, or most intriguing, to read about after each session. You may need to provide the student some guidance on where to look for the answer. Have the student prepare a brief summary of what was learned from the reading assignment. Don't forget to review the homework assignments with your student. Occasionally students need guidance from the clinical preceptor about choosing an appropriate question. For more advanced students, homework assignments become an opportunity to build skills in evidence-based medicine.

Finally, we should consider the importance of what our students learn from observing us, or from our role modeling. Role modeling is implicit – good role models inspire and teach while carrying out other tasks (Jochemsen-van der Leeuw et al. 2013). The language that we use and the stories that we tell are a powerful means of communicating professional values (Stern and Papdakis 2006). Think about what students learn when we describe a patient as "a good patient" or "a difficult patient". Our stories can reveal how we struggle to meet the highest standards of professional behavior – succeeding in most cases and yet sometimes failing (Bryden et al. 2010).

In order to help our students learn from our role modeling, we need to make what is implicit explicit. Reflective practice begins with being aware of yourself – your clinical knowledge and skills, your attitudes, and your weaknesses. You also need to be conscious of the attitudes and behaviors that you would like your students to develop. By talking through events you help students to pay attention to professional behaviors. You demonstrate how you want them to use what you have modeled to guide their own actions. Good role modeling can motivate students by creating a positive environment for learning and improving.

Summary

In this chapter, you have been introduced to teaching skills related to each of the key phases of teaching in clinical settings: planning for teaching, teaching during the clinical encounter, and reflecting on the clinical experience. Discuss the goals and expectations of the rotation – and the objective of each clinical encounter – with your student. Use effective questioning skills to promote your student's clinical judgment and problem solving skills. Explicitly demonstrate communication skills, clinical skills, and professional behaviors. Make frequent observations of your student's performance in each of these areas. Give regular constructive feedback. Spend time with your student reflecting on his clinical experiences. Enjoy the satisfaction of teaching students and contributing to their professional development.

References

Alguire PC, Dewitt DE, Pinsky LE, Ferenchick GS (2008) Teaching in your office: a guide to instructing medical students and residents, 2nd edn. American College of Physicians, Philadelphia

Bowen JL (2006) Educational strategies to promote clinical diagnostic reasoning. N Engl J Med 355:2217–2225

Bryden P, Ginsburg S, Kurabi B, Ahmed N (2010) Professing professionalism: are we our own worst enemy? Faculty members' experiences of teaching and evaluating professionalism in medical education at one school. Acad Med 85:1025–1034

Connell KJ, Bordage G, Chang RW, Howard BA, Sinacore J (1999) Measuring the promotion of thinking during precepting encounters in outpatient settings. Acad Med 74(10 suppl):S10–S12

Fromme HB, Bhansali P, Singhal G, Yudkowsky R, Humphrey H, Harris I (2010) The qualities and skills of exemplary pediatric hospitalist educators: a qualitative study. Acad Med 85:1905–1913

Hatem CJ, Searle NS, Gunderman R, Krane NK, Perkowski L, Schutze GE, Steinert Y (2011) The educational attributes and responsibilities of effective medical educators. Acad Med 86:474–480

Hewson MG, Little ML (1998) Giving feedback in medical education: verification of recommended techniques. J Gen Intern Med 13:111–116

Irby DM (1992) How attending physicians make instructional decisions when conducting teaching rounds. Acad Med 67:630–638

Jochemsen-van der Leeuw HGA, van Dijk N, van Etten-Jamaludin FS, Wieringa-Waard M (2013) The attributes of the clinical trainer as a role model: a systematic review. Acad Med 88:26–34

Neher JO, Gordon KC, Meyer B, Stevens N (1992) A five-step "microskills" model of clinical teaching. J Am Board Fam Pract 5:419–424

Peyton JWR (1998) The learning cycle. In: Peyton JMR (ed) Teaching and learning in medical practice. Manticore Europe Limited, Rickmansworth

Sachdeva AK (1996) Use of effective feedback to facilitate adult learning. J Cancer Educ 11:106–118

Stern DT, Papadakis M (2006) The developing physician – becoming a professional. N Engl J Med 355:1794–1799

Sutkin G, Wagner E, Harris I, Schiffer R (2008) What makes a good clinical teacher in medicine? Rev Lit Acad Med 83:452–466

Wilkerson L, Sarkin RT (1998) Arrows in the quiver: evaluation of a workshop on ambulatory teaching. Acad Med 73(10 suppl):S67–S69

Wolpaw TM, Wolpaw DR, Papp KK (2003) SNAPPS: a learner-centered model for outpatient education. Acad Med 78:893–898

Yudkowsky R, Otaki J, Lowenstein T, Riddle J, Nishigori H, Bordage G (2009) A hypothesis-driven physical examination learning and assessment procedure for medical students: initial validity evidence. Med Educ 43:729–740

For Further Reading

Wearne S, Dornan T, Teunissen PW, Skinner T (2012) General practitioners as supervisors in postgraduate clinical education: an integrative review. Med Educ 46:1161–1173

This literature review of clinical supervision in graduate medical education describes the intertwined clinical and educational roles of supervisors. Educational activities within the supervisory relationship should provide flexible and personal support to meet residents' learning needs and should also be appropriately challenging

Aagaard E, Teherani A, Irby DM (2004) Effectiveness of the one-minute preceptor model for diagnosing the patient and the learner: proof of concept. Acad Med 79:42–49

Irby DM, Aagaard E, Teherani A (2004) Teaching points identified by preceptors observing one-minute preceptor and traditional preceptor encounters. Acad Med 79:50–55

Salerno SM, O'Malley PG, Pangaro LN, Wheeler GA, Moores LK, Jackson JL (2002) Faculty development seminars based on the one-minute preceptor improve feedback in the ambulatory setting. J Gen Intern Med 17:779–787
These papers provide evidence for the effectiveness of the one-minute preceptor model presented in this chapter. In the first two papers listed above, preceptors viewed video-recordings of encounters in which the one-minute preceptor model was being used. Preceptors observing the videos rated the encounters as more effective than those in which the one-minute preceptor model was not used. Observers noted that teaching points using the one-minute preceptor model included a broader differential diagnosis, more discussion of the natural presentation of disease and of further diagnostic evaluation. Salerno and colleagues reported that participation in one-minute preceptor workshops increased the quality of feedback provided to students and preceptor satisfaction with teaching encounters
Wolpaw T, Papp KK, Bordage G (2009) Using SNAPPS to facilitate the expression of clinical reasoning and uncertainties: a randomized comparison group trial. Acad Med 84:517–524
Wolpaw T, Coté L, Papp KK, Bordage G (2012) Student uncertainties drive teaching during case presentations: more so with SNAPPS. Acad Med 87:1210–1217
These papers provide evidence for the effectiveness of the SNAPPS model. Compared with students who were not trained to use the SNAPPS model, students who were trained to use SNAPPS provided more concise case summaries, included more diagnoses in their differentials, provided better justifications for their differential diagnoses, and asked more questions or expressed more uncertainties – all without significantly increasing case presentation time. When students expressed uncertainties, their preceptors responded with teaching aligned to meet the students' learning needs
Archer JC (2010) State of the science in health professions education: effective feedback. Med Educ 44:101–108
Archer presents a critique of the current literature on feedback related to health professions education. He argues for the creation of a "culture of feedback" based upon promoting a dialog between teacher and student, facilitating self-monitoring of behavior by the student, and embedding feedback explicitly in all teaching activities
Rudolph JW, Simon R, Dufrense RL, Raemer DB (2006) There's no such thing as "nonjudgmental" debriefing: a theory and method for debriefing with good judgment. Simul Healthc 1:49–55
Rudolph and colleagues describe the "advocacy-inquiry" model of debriefing. In this model of reflective practice, debriefing is a conversation which teacher discloses her expert judgments about a student's performance while also eliciting and exploring the student's assumptions about the situation and reasons for acting as he did

Chapter 8
Teaching with Simulation

Cate Nicholas

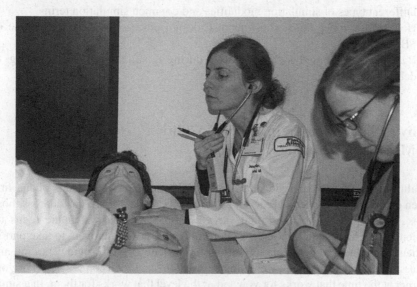

Abstract Simulation based medical education (SBME) imitates real healthcare encounters to enable learners to practice and receive feedback in a safe, supported learning environment. SBME can be used to improve competence and performance in clinical skills and procedures, communication skills and teamwork, patient management and decision-making. When used thoughtfully and carefully, simulation can be a transformational learning experience. Medical educators can create effective simulations when they are based on learning theories and evidence-based strategies.

C. Nicholas, Ed.D., MS-PA (✉)
Clinical Simulation Laboratory, Fletcher Allen Health Care/University
of Vermont, College of Medicine, Rowell 237, 106 Carrigan Dr.,
Burlington, VT 05404-00687, USA
e-mail: cate.nicholas@uvm.edu

K.N. Huggett and W.B. Jeffries (eds.), *An Introduction to Medical Teaching*,
DOI 10.1007/978-94-017-9066-6_8, © Springer Science+Business Media Dordrecht 2014

Introduction

Simulation based medical education (SBME) is a teaching strategy used to replicate real healthcare encounters in which learners practice and receive feedback within a safe, supported learning environment. SBME can be used to improve competence and performance in clinical skills and procedures, communication skills and teamwork, patient management and decision-making. When used thoughtfully and carefully, simulation can be a transformational learning experience (Anderson et al. 2008). Medical educators can create effective simulations when they are based on learning theories and evidence-based strategies. This chapter will help you understand:

1. Why SBME is an important addition to medical education
2. How SBME leads to effective learning
3. Different types of simulation modalities and common simulation terms
4. How to use a step-by-step instructional design process for the effective use of SBME
5. Basic evidence-based strategies used during a simulation from briefing to debriefing

Why Is Simulation an Important Addition to Medical Education?

Healthcare and healthcare education are rapidly changing. The needs of the first often do not meet the needs of the second, and vice versa. SBME can address those gaps. Decreased length of hospital stays combined with a systematic focus on patient safety has resulted in fewer opportunities for novice learners to take part in patient care. Integrating simulation into your curriculum will provide learning and assessment on demand, i.e., by creating simulations that focus on the needs of your learner at the time that works for you and at the level that works for them. In a simulated clinical environment, learners practice and reflect on what occurred during the scenario. Actions taken during simulation that lead to poor outcomes can be discussed during the debriefing and no one is harmed in the process (Gordon et al. 2004; Ziv et al. 2006).

Increased clinical productivity demands of healthcare faculty have reduced time for bedside teaching. The result is learners with decreased competence in clinical skills (e.g., performing the cardiac exam with the inability to recognize common heart murmurs). Simulation can overcome this deficit by teaching and assessing skills outside of the patient care arena. For example, simulation exercises that employ a concept called deliberate practice (repetitive practice of cognitive and psychomotor skills linked to specific and immediate feedback and assessment), have been shown to be superior to experience in the clinical setting (Ericsson 2008; Butter et al. 2010). This is key to developing competence for clinical skills and procedures.

Table 8.1 Benefits of SBME teaching strategy

1. It is based on level and needs of learner
2. Learning and assessment available as needed for the curriculum; not dependent on patient census
3. Allows time for immediate and purposeful feedback and practice (deliberate practice)
4. No risk to patients and learners
5. Increases knowledge and skill acquisition through repetitive practice and reflection
6. Transfer of knowledge and skills to real world is increased

In summary, developing simulation using deliberate practice that is tailored to the level and needs of your learner is superior to relying on the chance that the kind of patient problem your learner needs to see will present itself in the clinical setting. Table 8.1 summarizes the benefits of SBME as a teaching strategy.

How Does SBME Lead to Effective Learning?

To appreciate how SBME is an effective teaching strategy, it is important to understand how students learn from the simulation process. The process begins with linking learning objectives to an appropriate simulation activity. The learning objectives define the **desired performance**. The learners go through the simulation while being observed by the faculty. The difference between the desired performance and the **actual performance** in the simulation is the called the **performance gap** (Rudolph et al. 2008). During the **debriefing**, with the help of an expert facilitator, the learners identify which actions were taken during the simulation and reflect on the underlying reasons for the performance gap. This process allows the learner to think back to discover what thought or assumption may have contributed to the gap. Reflection requires the facilitator and the learner to return to the simulation experience, attend to the feelings associated with the experience (the emotional component), and reevaluate the experience (Schon 1987). If the facilitator has created and maintained a safe and supported learning environment during this process, the learner will be ready to then accept and integrate new knowledge, skills and behaviors in future simulation and in the clinical setting (**learning outcomes**). Figure 8.1 describes the simulation educational process.

Medical Simulators

Simulation works best when incorporated within an existing curriculum. The choice of simulators is driven by the curriculum, not the other way around. Understanding which simulators are needed for your curriculum prior to purchase saves time and resources. Medical Simulation includes human simulation and non-human simulation.

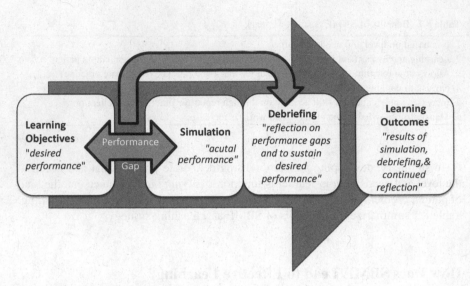

Fig. 8.1 Simulation education process

Non-human Simulation

Simulators are devices that mimic a real patient, part of the human body, system or process, and are capable of interacting with the learner (Cooper and Taqueti 2008; Gaba 2004). The number and types of simulators available grows every year while the costs continue to go down. The possibilities of how to integrate non-human simulators into your curriculum are endless and limited by your imagination and resources. High fidelity mannequins can be used in basic sciences lectures to demonstrate principles of physiology. Task trainers can be used for central line insertion instruction for residents, or Foley catheter models can be used to address patient safety issues. Complex task trainers like Harvey® The Cardiopulmonary Patient Simulator can be used to create a longitudinal cardiovascular curriculum for undergraduate, graduate and CME. Computer based simulation and virtual reality may allow you to overcome some of the logistical challenges of interprofessional education. Table 8.2 reviews different types of non-human simulation modalities.

Human Simulation

As you read through the simulation literature, you will find many different terms to describe humans in simulation: standardized patients, simulated patients, simulated participants, embedded participants, actors, simulated actors, and confederates. The international simulation community has yet to come to a consensus on terminology. This chapter will define two terms, standardized/simulated patient and confederate.

Table 8.2 Non-human simulation modalities

Types	Description
Complex task trainers	Complex computer generated environments which provide opportunity to practice complex skills. These programs can be found on screen-based programs or within partial task trainers like. Harvey® The Cardiopulmonary Patient Simulator or other devices that simulate endoscopic devices and robotic surgical trainers, ultrasound trainers or arthroscopic trainers. Some of these trainers contain haptic systems which provide the learner with tactile or pressure sensation to increase the fidelity of the simulation
Full-scale mannequin	Life-sized robot (adults, children, infants, birthing mothers) that mimics various functions of the human body, including respiration, cardiac rhythms, and pulsation. The low-fidelity mannequins are used to practice simple physical maneuvers or procedures like CPR. The high-fidelity mannequins have responsive airways, and pupils, and physiologic responses to certain medications and interventions. These mannequins can be used for complex, team training scenarios or can be used for demonstration of basic sciences principles in large group settings. Mannequins come as adults, children, birthing mothers, and preemies to newborns and young children
Part or partial task trainer	Physical model that simulates a subset of physiologic function to include normal and abnormal anatomy. As the name implies, these trainers are used to teach specific tasks. Examples include intubation heads, IV arm and Foley catheter models
Virtual reality	Programs, exclusively computer-based, that allow learners to interview, examine, diagnose, and treat patients in realistic clinical scenarios. May also be used to train and assess clinical reasoning skills and decision making

A Standardized/Simulated Patient (SP) is a person trained to portray a patient scenario, or an actual patient using their own history and physical exam findings, for the instruction, assessment, or practice of a health care provider's communication and/or examining skills. In the health and medical sciences, SPs are used to provide a safe and supportive environment conducive for learning or for standardized assessment. SPs can serve as practice models, or participate in sophisticated assessment and feedback of provider abilities or services. Here are some of the ways to use SPs in the curriculum.

- Case based teaching scenarios for one-on-one or small group teaching
- Demonstrations in front of large groups
- Psychiatric mental health cases
- Teaching communication and interpersonal skills (giving bad news or sad news)
- Teaching history and interviewing skills
- Teaching patient education and counseling skills
- Teaching physical exam skills

Two types of speciality trained SPs are Gynecological Teaching Associates (GTAs) and Male Urogenital Associates (MUTAs). GTAs are women who are specifically trained to teach, assess, and provide feedback to learners about the

Table 8.3 Humans in simulation

Type	Description
Standardized/Simulated Patient (SP)	A person trained to portray a patient scenario, or an actual patient using their own history and physical exam findings, for the instruction, assessment, or practice of communication and/or examining skills of a health care provider
Gynecological Teaching Associate (GTA)	Women who are specifically trained to teach assess and provide feedback to learners about the breast, pelvic and rectal exams
Male Urogenital Associate (MUTA)	Men who are specifically trained to teach, assess and provide feedback to learners about the urogenital and rectal exams
Confederate	A person who supplies additional information within the simulation and to help the learners navigate an unfamiliar simulation environment if needed

breast, pelvic and rectal exams. MUTAs are men who are specifically trained to teach, assess and provide feedback to learners about the urogenital and rectal exams. Both use their bodies to teach and they provide a safe and supported learning environment while addressing communication skills necessary to provide a patient centered exam.

SPs and mannequins can be used together in mixed modality simulations. The SP can play the part of the any family member of the mannequin. Some faculty have trained SPs to play other professionals within the team e.g., doctors, nurse, or respiratory technician. Training is required for an SP to play a participant in a simulation with a mannequin to meet the level of realism required for the scenario. Hybrid simulation is when a SP has a part or partial task trainer attached to them. For example, an SP can have an IV arm attached to them or they can have an IM pad attached to their arm.

Another role for a human in a simulation is called a confederate. The confederate role is sometimes confused with the SP role. While confederates also require careful scripting and training, their primary functions are to supply additional information within the simulation and to can help the learners navigate an unfamiliar simulation environment if needed. The role of the confederate is often played by a simulation technician who knows the simulation environment well, a faculty member who is well versed in the simulation, or another faculty member from a different discipline whose content knowledge is necessary for the simulation to run smoothly. Table 8.3 reviews definitions for humans in used simulation.

Planning Stages of Simulation Based Medical Curriculum Design

Before you begin planning, acquaint yourself with the simulation resources at your institution. The size and scope of your simulation program are important factors to consider. The faculty and staff are critical partners in developing your simulation.

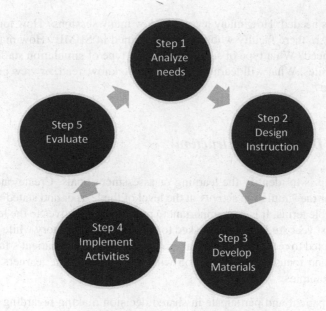

Fig. 8.2 ADDIE curriculum design model (Dick and Carey 1996)

They are your content experts when it comes to simulation and standardized patient education and you might consider including them on your planning team from the very beginning.

Quality SBME starts with good instructional design. A common instructional design model that can be adapted to SBME curriculum design is called **"ADDIE"**: **A**nalyze needs, **D**esign instruction, **D**evelop materials, **I**mplement Activities and **E**valuate participants and program's effectiveness (Dick and Carey 1996) (Fig. 8.2).

Step One: Needs Analysis

You can do this before you meet with the simulation staff or they can walk you through a needs analysis during a planning session. Questions to answer during this step:

- Learning Need: Is this a learning activity? Is this a formative or summative assessment? Are you addressing learning or skills gaps? Is this a new initiative or a research project?
- Learner: What is the level of the learner on the medical education continuum? What is the level of the learner for knowledge, skills or behavior being taught (novice to expert)? Are you working within a single discipline or with multidisciplinary program? Is this an interprofessional project?

- Resources needed: How many learners? How many sessions? How long is each session? Are there faculty who need to be trained in SBME? How many rooms will you need? What type of simulation? What type of simulation staff support?
- Pre-requisites: What will learners be required to know, read, or view prior to the simulation?

Step Two: Design the Instruction

The next step is to identify the learning or assessment goals. Create one to three objectives for the simulation activity at the level of the learner and stated in specific and measurable terms. It is very important to match the objectives to the level of the learner. A first year student may be asked to obtain a patient history while a resident will be expected to recognize a medical error and disclose to a patient's family. The complexity and focus of the simulation will vary based on the learners. Here are additional examples:

- Assess a patient and participate in shared decision making regarding treatment options
- Deliver sad or bad news
- Evaluate and triage mass casualty incidents
- Insert a Foley catheter
- Insert an central line
- Plan and prepare for discharge with the family and healthcare team (MD, nurse, OT, PT and home health care agency)
- Recognize an imminent crisis situation

Step Three: Design Materials

Decide if you want to create a new simulation-based learning or assessment activity or adapt an existing one. Consider the type of simulation modality needed. Sometimes what you might have thought was most appropriate as a mannequin simulation will work best with a SP or will work even better as a mixed modality. The addition of an SP as a family member or other participant can add the human dimension to your simulation. On the other hand, as your SP cannot simulate abnormal vital signs, you can add some of the simulator's technology for a more authentic clinical scenario.

Seek out an experienced simulation/SP educator to help you adapt an existing simulation activity to meet your needs so you do not need to start from scratch. Many low and high fidelity mannequins will come with simulation scenarios ready to use. Many cases can be found in the medical literature, via online searches and from simulation societies. If you cannot locate the appropriate activity, make use of a template to help organize your thinking and create a reusable asset for yourself and others. Examples of such templates have been compiled in the curriculum repository MedEdPortal, and links to them can be found in the references at the end of this chapter. You can base your scenarios on a real patient case, critical incident report or patient safety goals so long as it is developed at the level of the learner and linked to your objectives. Achieving a good balance between developing scenarios to address specific learning objectives and allowing for unplanned moments to emerge (teachable moments) is critical in simulation (Alinier 2011).

Details of the simulation scenario/SP case: You are writing your scenario/case for two audiences: (1) the learners who need to understand what is expected of them and (2) the simulation technician(s) who will be operating the mannequin or the SP who will be portraying the role. Thus, for each situation you need to provide an introduction to the simulation to the learner and a simulation design/SP case and logistical information to the simulation staff.

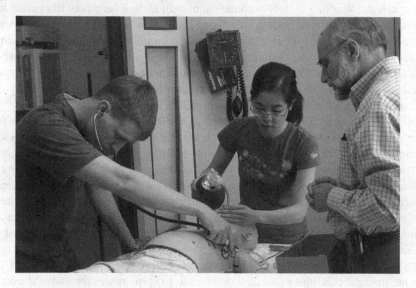

Let's start with the simulation scenario.

Introduction to the scenario: Learners are usually provided with a limited amount of information about the patient prior to the beginning of the encounter in the form of a "hand off" or nurse's report or EMT report. The information can be provided orally or with written instructions based on the level of the learner or situation.

Scenario design: The details of the scenario provide the faculty and the simulation technician with details about how the case should run and how the mannequin should respond in certain circumstances.

1. What information the learners are provided or given freely if they ask
2. What the learners must ascertain during the simulation
3. Branch Points based on the action or inaction of the learner(s)

You must decide on the end point of the simulation but remember it may change with each group of learners based on their actions and your observations. Once engaged in the encounter, the scenario needs to have the flexibility to adapt to the action of the participants by either speeding up or slowing down the patient's symptom arc. If standardized participants play family members or staff, they can adapt the scenario in the moment as needed.

You can use preprogrammed settings on the mannequin to progress the case or you can control the mannequin manually based on the observed response of the learners. The choice is a matter of preference based on your experience, comfort, the scenario at hand, and working relationship with the simulation technician. Remember one advantage of simulation is that you can adjust a basic scenario to the level of the learner. For example, you can use the scenario of a patient presenting with an acute abdominal pain for first-year medical learners today and with some fine tuning you can run the same patient case tomorrow for first-year internal medicine residents. Working closely with the simulation technician who will operate the mannequin will help guarantee a successful simulation for you and your learners. Some faculty eventually learn to run the mannequin and the session at the same time. Only you will be able to make that decision once you have become more experienced in simulation. The details of the scenario will dictate which type of mannequin you will be able to use although sometimes you will need to adjust your scenario to the type of mannequin that is available in your simulation center.

Now, let's look at SP case development. The SP case is the building block for your program. Once you know how to develop one case, you can go on to develop a case bank from which you can build multi-station exams. If you create a good system to categorize your cases, you will be able to reuse them for different levels of learners and different types of learners more easily. There are many different approaches to developing cases. Some faculty members base their cases on real patients they have encountered, while some create fictional cases. Regardless, cases should be linked to the instructional goals and objectives. The case material is developed for the SP to memorize. Case material should be written in language that the SP can understand. SPs might sometimes be provided with background on chronic medical conditions included in the case to help answer questions if asked. Scripts become more detailed as the learners and the instructional and assessment goals become more advanced.

The case material not only contains factual information about the patient but also about affect and emotional reactions based on learners' actions. When writing a case the basic idea is to give the standardized patient more information about the patient they are portraying then they will ever be asked about by the learner. To be as authentic as possible, the SP has to know these patients as well as they know themselves so they could respond to any question asked of them by any learner as this patient might respond without giving an answer that might inadvertently mislead the learner. When you are creating the cases, be sure to specify if there are any specific body types or physical requirement, specific dress or props that should be present. For example, if you are writing an acute abdomen case, the SPs who are hired for the case cannot have had an appendectomy or any abdomen surgery that might mislead the learner.

Table 8.4 Goals and objectives of SP training

1. Realistically portray the patient as written in the scenario
2. Respond to the learner appropriately no matter what the learner says or does
3. Observe and recall learner performance and accurately complete checklist
4. Provide effective written or verbal feedback to the learner
5. Standardize to other SPs in same role
6. Do 1–5 repeatedly in a teaching or assessment session

Once you have written your SP case, you must pick right the SP to portray a particular patient case. Matching the SP to the case is as important as having a well-written case and training materials in the first place. Choose an SP whose profile is as close to the case description as possible. Ethnicity, age and gender are the three main characteristics to consider. **A word about age**: it does not matter what the SPs actual age is as long as they look within the age range of the patient profile. Selecting SPs who can play the same age makes exam administration easier as the age on the door instructions to the students can all be the same, and it keeps the student experience as close to standard as possible. The gender or ethnicity in a case can be varied, depending on the case goal and objectives.

Train all SPs who are doing the same case as a group to ensure their understanding of this patient, answer questions about the patient profile and share suggestions for portrayal. Standardized patients are very helpful in discovering problems in the case and bringing the patient to life. Together the instructor and patients reach consensus on how the patient is to be played, and how the patient will respond to the learner. In this way, we standardize the SPs in the way they think and present the patient to the learners.

SPs must be trained to appropriately and accurately respond to questions about the patient's problems. They must consistently reproduce any emotional and/or physical pain the patient is feeling while they are observing the learner's behavior. They also need to accurately recall those behaviors to complete a checklist and or provide the learner with feedback over and over again.

(Wallace 2007). Once you have trained the case to performance level, ask another faculty who is familiar with the case content to observe the SPs to validate the performance and correct the portrayal. Table 8.4 reviews the goals of SP training.

An equally important component is the logistics of the simulation. If you are doing this in a simulation center, work with the staff early to carefully plan the simulation. Attention to detail during planning will help the staff know how to prepare for your simulation.

Elements to consider:

- Schedule: day, time, and frequency
- Specific patient rooms: inpatient, outpatient, operating room, emergency/trauma room

- Room amenities: phones, access to bathrooms, ability to monitor and record video
- Room set up: medical equipment, code carts, materials and supplies, EHR etc.
- Handouts and materials: have adequate copies ready to distribute to learners on day of the simulation
- Mannequin/SP: initial set up position, presentation, dress, Moulage (e.g., make up, blood), props etc.
- Access to conference rooms and debriefing rooms

Step Four: Implement Activities

Once you have made all of your decisions, the mannequins are programmed, and the SPs are trained, the stage is set for a dress rehearsal. The simulation technicians, standardized patients, simulator, and faculty involved in the scenario should be brought into the simulation setting. The simulation should be run for a group of learners similar to your target group: a simulation of the simulation! Debriefing the dress rehearsal will be very valuable. You will learn what you have forgotten to consider in the scenario script, what props you have left out, what does not flow, what a staff member does not understand or where a fellow faculty member is in disagreement. Even though the rehearsal takes time and resources, your simulation will be greatly improved. The less familiar you are with simulation, the more important the dress rehearsal is.

Showtime: After you have completed your preparation, conducted a dress rehearsal and/or piloted the simulation, you will be feeling confident about the simulation going smoothly. This is when it is important to remember that you are working with computers and humans, which often do not perform as expected. Even if you checked the simulator 10 min ago, there could be a problem the moment you need it to work. You need to plan for what you will do when the mannequin is not working or the trained SP is unavailable or the faculty member you were counting on gets called away. What is your back up plan? Remember you work in health care or in the laboratory; you live with uncertainty every day so use that experience and make it work for you.

Before the simulation, make sure the learners have received clear instructions and written materials to help them prepare for the session. Everyone will be anxious. Any steps you can take to reassure them as to where they should be, and at what time, will go a long way to help them be ready to learn.

There are three components of any simulation:

1. Briefing
2. Simulation
3. Debriefing

Each is as important as the other. You have spent time and money planning the simulation. Equal attention must be paid to the briefing and the debriefing preparation and execution.

Briefing: Make Room for Learning

You need to prepare your learners to feel safe to engage in reflection and self-examination. Therefore the briefing before the scenario is crucial. Here are ten steps that can build trust among you and your learners:

1. Welcome each of the learners as they enter the conference/briefing room.
2. Introduce yourself and simulation staff (but not the SPs).
3. Introduce participants (if unfamiliar to each other).
4. Discuss care and comfort issues (restrooms, breaks etc.).
5. Review course objectives and format of the simulation.
6. Provide a tour in the setting of the simulation and let the learners explore and ask as many questions as needed for them to feel as prepared as possible.
7. Discuss and agree to the "Fiction Contract." This means that the learner willingly agrees to suspend disbelief and you will do your best to make the simulation as real as possible with the understanding that while mannequins are not humans and SPs are not real patients, much can be learned that will be helpful in a real world setting (Dieckmann et al. 2007).
8. State that the learning team (learners and faculty/staff) will provide each other with a safe and supported learning environment. This means the environment will remain predictable and secure. During debriefing, instructors will help learners explore without risk and learners will engage in reflection and share their best thinking.
9. The learners agree to confidentiality and if it is your policy can sign a confidentiality agreement.
10. Make sure there are no questions or outstanding issues prior to beginning the simulation.

Simulation

For standardized patient cases, instructions are usually posted on the examination room door and provide the patient's name, age, sex, and chief complaint. Based on the goals and objectives and the level of the learner, the door instructions then tell the learner what would they would be expected to do and how much time they have with the patient.

While the simulation is taking place, you may have a choice of observing from inside the room or from a remote location (e.g., a control or conference room, hallway through a window, etc.), based on the setting or goals of the scenario. If you have a choice and it does not affect the goals of the scenario, I recommend that you choose the remote option. Learners will then have more autonomy to act and will therefore have a better learning experience. You will have great opportunity to observe and gather data for debriefing from behind the one-way mirror or electronic monitor. Having your objectives in front of you and jotting down observations associated with each of them will be helpful for debriefing. Pay careful attention during the transitions that you have built into the scenario.

When the simulation is completed, go into the room and simply say "The simulation is over." Often the learners will be so engaged in caring for the "patients" that

Table 8.5 Tips for using recording to your advantage for debriefing

1. Become familiar with the equipment
   a. Fast forward
   b. Book marking
   c. Focus on 2–4 segments as springboards for discussion
2. Segments that are often best used for discussion are:
   a. Near the beginning
   b. When there is a change in vital signs
   c. If you have scripted something to happen
   d. Before a call for help
   e. When help arrives
   f. If a correct or incorrect diagnosis or procedure is started
   g. 3–5 min into the scenario

you will have to reassure them that it is okay for them to leave. In this case it is helpful if the simulation technicians move close to the mannequins or the SPs to take over from the learners. As soon as the learners begin to leave the simulation room they will begin to debrief with each other.

If you have the ability to record the session, research shows video is a powerful learning tool that will be helpful in the next stage, debriefing. Table 8.5 lists tips for using recording to your advantage during a debriefing.

If you are debriefing as a team, it is best when you can take a few minutes to decide how to structure the focus of the debriefing. This is especially important if something happened during the simulation that you did not expect and you want to be sure to cover it during the debriefing. You will have to do this in a short period of time as you don't want to miss too much of the group's post scenario auto-debrief.

Basics of Debriefing

Debriefing is where learning takes place as students reflect on the process and results of the simulation. The goal of the debriefing is to sustain or improve future performance by methodically reviewing what happened and why. The learners need to feel they are in a safe, supported learning environment so they can reflect on habits, techniques or approaches and evaluate their decision making. This debriefing process will allow them to accept and assimilate new knowledge, behaviors, techniques and approaches.

There are different phases to debriefing and styles of facilitation (Fanning and Gaba 2007). The initial phase is to ask participants to share how they are feeling and to describe, in their own words, what happened and what they did. The second phase is to reflect on and analyze the experience and the third phase is to generalize the experience and apply the lessons learned to real life events. In the second phase of debriefing different techniques are employed. Some facilitators ask specific ques-

Table 8.6 Elements of good debriefing

Elements of good debriefing	The debriefer
1. Establish an engaging learning environment	Welcomes learners and attends to logistical details
	Introduces learning objectives and outcomes
	Orients to the simulation environment and clarifies limitations of the simulation methods
	Establishes confidentiality
	Obtains agreement that everyone will be respectful of each other's perspectives
	Assures participants of physical and psychological safety
2. Maintain an engaging learning environment	Maintains participants' physical and psychological safety
	Helps participants move into, stay in and move out of the simulation
3. Structure the debriefing in an organized way	Has participants:
	Share their reactions
	Describe events from their perspectives
	Reflect/analyze on what went well and what could have gone better based on the objectives
	Close performance gaps
	Summarize key points made and take home messages
4. Facilitate engaging discussions	Uses specific examples of what was done well and not done based on objectives for discussion
	Engages all participants in discussion through verbal and nonverbal techniques
	Recognizes when participants are upset and works with them
	Uses audio/video replay if available
5. Identify and explore performance gaps (difference between actual performance and expected performance)	Provides direct feedback on performance gaps
	Explores reason for gap by working with group to identify what "mental models" or frames (assumptions, feelings, goals, knowledge base or situation awareness) learners were working with during the simulation that led to those the actions and results
6. Help trainees achieve and/or sustain good future performance	Helps close the performance gap through discussion and teaching
	Meets the objectives of the session
	Shows knowledge of the subject

tions about certain actions, or let the group lead the way. Some facilitators will use the plus/delta technique: participants are asked to place all behaviors or actions they would change in the delta column and place all the examples of good behaviors or actions in the plus column for discussion. How much the debriefer needs to facilitate is dependent on the group and the skill of the debriefer. Ideally, you want the group to learn how to debrief themselves with minimum facilitation. The debriefer provides guided facilitation only when necessary to be sure the objectives are met.

Regardless of the specific debriefing method used for reflection after the simulation, Breet-Fleeger et al. (2012) identified six elements of good debriefing practices. In Table 8.6 you will find elements of good debriefing adapted to include all types of debriefing styles and methods.

Table 8.7 Tips for working
with learners who break the
"fiction contract"

Agree with them
Be sympathetic- don't argue
Redirect to a productive discussion about real world setting
Clinical discussion to reestablish comfort

Debriefing usually takes 30–45 min based on the learning objectives and other learning that may have emerged from simulation. The debriefer and the learners share responsibility during the debriefing session, which should be reviewed and agreed to during the briefing session.

If at any time during debrief you have a participant who was unable to suspend disbelief and has broken the "fiction contract" and you are getting complaints about the realism, be sympathetic and don't argue. Redirect the conversation to a productive discussion using real world examples. "What CAN we learn from this experience that would be helpful in a real world setting?" "Has anything like this happened in a real clinical setting?" If so, give a personal example. Using a clinical discussion often reestablishes comfort, (Rudolph et al. 2007) Table 8.7 review tips for how to work with learners who have trouble with simulation realism.

When the session is over, thank your learners for participating in the simulation and engaging in the debriefing. Make sure that there are no outstanding issues before ending and sending learners on their way.

Techniques to Facilitate Debriefings

Debriefing is an advanced skill and takes many sessions with feedback from fellow debriefers to improve. There are some techniques that you can use that will help your session run more smoothly as you improve your skills.

Make sure the room is arranged so everyone can see each other. If there are two debriefers (which is ideal) they should sit at the opposite end of the table. Be sure to make use active listening skills, verbal and nonverbal. Nod your head, make eye contact and be very aware of body language. Use echoing and reflective listening: repeat or rephrase the speaker's words back to the group. Be careful not to put your words into the learner's mouth and don't interrupt. Be sure to involve everyone. Invite them into the discussion by name. Ask a learner in the group to comment on something said by another member of the group. Be comfortable with silence. If there is no response to a question, give the learners time to think and then follow up with another question if no response. It is okay to allow and encourage the learners to talk and ask each other questions (Breet-Fleeger et al. 2012).

Even though you have outlined a set of learning objectives, learners will do unexpected things during simulation unrelated to the objectives (teachable moments) that you may want to use during debriefing. Learners will do something wonderfully clever, choose to do nothing at all or make a mistake you could never have anticipated. These should be discussed during debriefing as they add richness to the overall learning experience (Ziv et al. 2005).

Step Five: Evaluation

There are two areas to consider, one for the learner and one for the program.

Learner Assessment

Summative feedback provides information about learning in high stakes situations like course requirements, graduation requirements, certification or licensure. Summative assessment relies on careful planning. Many tools are available and shown to be valid in the setting in which they were developed. Retesting for validity for your learner and your setting may be required. Assuring your learners and other stakeholders of the reliability and validity of your simulation and defensible standard setting process for summative assessment is paramount to the credibility of your program (McGaghie 2011).

Formative assessment provides learner feedback for knowledge or skill improvement under low stakes conditions. After a simulation, we use debriefing to facilitate conversation among learners. They analyze their actions, thought processes, and emotional states to improve or sustain performance in future situations. The strength of simulation-based education lies with debriefing and the development of this reflective thought process. Schon (2003) defines reflection as a process that turns a person's experience into learning. During debriefing we ask learners to think back on what they did (reflection on action) in order to discover what might have contributed to an unexpected outcome. Boud et al. (1985) stressed that effective reflection on action requires the learner to return to the experience, attend to the feelings, and re-evaluate the experience. Research has shown this type of debriefing has improved performance and decreased clinical errors (Mamede et al. 2007).

Program Evaluation

Identify how the simulation activity/program will be assessed by learners to aid in ongoing quality improvement. Kirkpatrick (1994) developed four levels of evaluation for overall program effectiveness, which can be applied to simulation programs:

1. Reaction to the simulation experience: satisfaction, perception of program quality.
2. Learning: knowledge or skill acquisition/improvement or behavior change.
3. Behavior: application of knowledge/skill or behavior in the real world based on what was learned in simulation.
4. Outcome: long term impact on the learner, system, or organization as result of simulation.

It is vital that you evaluate every simulation session and debrief session. Decide when and how you want to get feedback from the learners about the simulation experience. Ideally you should leave some time at the end of the session for learners to complete the evaluation. If that is not possible they should complete the evaluation at a later date. For ongoing program improvement and feedback to your faculty, develop a form that provides similar information to allow for comparison.

Now it is your turn:

This chapter has given you the basic overview of:

1. How SBME addresses challenges faced by medical educators today
2. The instructional design process for SBME using ADDIE model
3. The steps of simulation from Briefing to Debriefing

There are two professional associations, The Association of Standardized Patient Educators http://aspeducators.org and The Society for Simulation in Health Care http://ssih.org, that offer yearly conferences and webinars in professional development workshops that will deepen your understanding of the knowledge, skills and behaviors needed to become an expert in SBME. The most challenging and most rewarding is the art of debriefing. While most of the attention and money is spent on the mannequins and the virtual hospitals, the actual learning takes place in classrooms and conference rooms in simulation centers around the world during debriefing. There is nothing more rewarding than being part of that transformative process. Just like your learners, you will want to do another simulation and debrief again and soon.

References

Alinier GA (2011) A guide for developing high fidelity simulation scenarios in healthcare education and continuing profession development. Simul Gaming 42:9–26

Anderson JM, Aylor ME, Leonard DT (2008) Instructional design dogma: creating planned learning experiences in simulation. J Crit Care 23:595–602

Boud D, Keogh R, Walker D (1985) Reflection: turning experience into learning. Kogan Page, London

Breet-Fleeger M, Rudolph J, Eppich W, Monuteaux M, Fleegler E, Cheng A, Simon R (2012) Debriefing assessment for simulation in healthcare: development and psychometric properties. Simul Healthc 7(5):288–294

Butter J, McGaghie WC, Cohen ER, Kaye M, Wayne DB (2010) Simulation-based mastery learning improves cardiac auscultation skills in medical learners. J Gen Intern Med 25(8):780–785

Cooper JB, Taqueti VR (2008) A brief history of the development of mannequin simulators for clinical education and training. Postgrad Med J 84:563–570

Dick W, Carey L (1996) The systematic design of instruction, 4th edn. Harper Collins College Publishers, New York

Dieckmann P, Gaba D, Rall M (2007) Deepening the theoretical foundations of patient simulation as social practice. Simul Healthc 2:183–193

Ericsson KA (2008) Deliberate practice and acquisition of expert performance: a general overview. Acad Emerg Med 15:988–994

Fanning RM, Gaba DM (2007) The role of debriefing in simulation based learning. Simul Healthc 2:1–11

Gaba DM (2004) The future vision of simulation in health care. Qual Saf Health Care 13 (Suppl 1):i2–i10

Gordon JA, Oriol ND, Cooper JB (2004) Bringing good teaching cases "to life": a simulator-based medical education service. Acad Med 79:23–27

Kirkpatrick DL (1994) Evaluating training effectiveness: the four levels. Bennett-Koehler, San Francisco

Mamede S, Schmidt JG, Rikers R (2007) Diagnostic errors and reflective practice in medicine. J Eval Clin Pract 13(1):138–145

McGaghie WC (2011) Use of simulation to assess competence and improve healthcare. Med Sci Educ 21(3S):261–263

Medical Simulation in Medical Education: Results of an AAMC Survey. Retrieved 23 April 2012 from https://www.aamc.org/download/259760/data/

Rudolph JW, Simon R, Raemer DB (2007) Which reality matters? Questions on the path to high engagement in healthcare simulation. Simul Healthc 2(3):161–163

Rudolph JW, Simon R, Raemer DB, Eppich WJ (2008) Debriefing as formative assessment: closing performance gaps in medical education. Acad Emerg Med 15:1010–1016

Schön D (1987) Educating the reflective practitioner. Jossey-Bass, San Francisco

Schon DA (2003) Educating the reflective practitioner: educating the reflective practitioner: towards a new design for teaching and learning in the professions. Teach Assess Clinic Pract: 323–325

Wallace P (2007) Coaching standardized patients for use in the assessment of clinical competence. Springer, New York

Ziv A, Ben-David S, Ziv M (2005) Simulation based medical education. An opportunity to learn from errors. Med Teach 27(3):193–199

Ziv A, Erez D, Munz Y, Vardi A, Barsuk D, Levine I, Benita S, Rubin O, Berkenstadt H (2006) The Israel center for medical simulation: a paradigm for cultural change in medical education. Acad Med 81:1091–1097

Chapter 9
Teaching with Practicals and Labs

Travis P. Webb, Carole S. Vetter, and Karen J. Brasel

Abstract Over the last 50 years, medical education has seen an increase in time devoted to didactic teaching and a significant decline in the amount of time devoted to laboratory teaching and learning. The reasons for this are multifaceted, and the end result is not only unfortunate but ignores sound educational and learning theory. However, recently health science schools are increasingly searching for ways to incorporate active learning strategies in their curricula. This chapter addresses that need and will help incorporate laboratory exercises into your teaching repertoire.

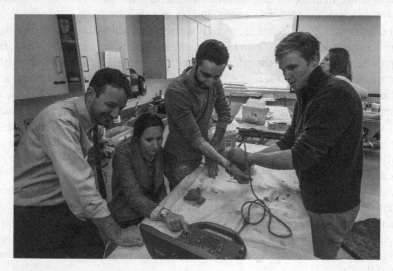

T.P. Webb, M.D., MHPE (✉) • K.J. Brasel, M.D., MPH
Department of Surgery-Trauma, Critical Care, Medical College of Wisconsin,
9200 W. Wisconsin Ave, Milwaukee, WI 53226, USA
e-mail: trwebb@mcw.edu; kbrasel@mcw.edu

C.S. Vetter, M.D.
Department of Orthopedics, Medical College of Wisconsin, Milwaukee, WI, USA
e-mail: cvetter@mcw.edu

K.N. Huggett and W.B. Jeffries (eds.), *An Introduction to Medical Teaching*,
DOI 10.1007/978-94-017-9066-6_9, © Springer Science+Business Media Dordrecht 2014

Introduction

Modern medical education has seen an increase in time devoted to didactic teaching and a significant decline in the amount of time devoted to laboratory teaching and learning. The reasons for this are multifaceted, and the end result is not only unfortunate but ignores sound educational and learning theory. Many leaders in education recognize the negative consequences of relying on passive learning and have taken measures to increase interactive learning opportunities. However, hands-on laboratory teaching remains a small portion of most medical school curricula. We hope that the fact that you are reading this chapter indicates your interest in laboratory teaching and that you will find the information helpful as you incorporate laboratory exercises into your teaching repertoire.

Benefits of Laboratory Teaching

Laboratory teaching is one form of active learning, or the process of having students engage in an activity that forces them to reflect on ideas and how they are using those ideas. Knowledge is gained through a cycle of hands on experience with reflection guided to conceptualization and then returning to application. When complemented by self-assessment the student's understanding and skill are further enhanced.

Laboratory teaching requires a change from teacher-focused lecturing to student-focused learning. Far from relieving the instructor from responsibility, laboratory teaching can increase the effort and time required of teachers, at least early in the transition from didactic lectures. The benefit? Increased student interest, attention, and knowledge retention. Most, although not all, studies suggest enhanced information transfer as evidenced by improved exam scores compared to students taught in didactic curricula. In addition, the majority of laboratory exercises are group learning events. This facilitates better solutions to problems, increased mastery of conceptual reasoning and retention compared to learning alone. These exercises can also develop critical skills in communication and team dynamics.

Laboratory teaching is often an opportunity to involve clinicians early in the science curriculum. The potential advantages are great—the students' education is enhanced by participating in an active learning exercise, the basic scientists are rewarded by interested and motivated students who can apply core concepts, and the clinicians benefit from early exposure to students, thus increasing student interest in their field.

Examples of Laboratory Teaching

Before we get into the nuts and bolts of how to conduct successful laboratory learning opportunities, here are a few examples of places they might be incorporated into an undergraduate medical curriculum. A word of caution—time in an undergraduate curriculum is scarce, and the addition of hours to an already overloaded schedule is often impossible. However, some schools have been able to use well designed laboratory teaching to decrease overall curriculum time. Creativity and cooperation among instructors along the basic science and clinical continuum are required to determine whether laboratory teaching is feasible, whether it can supplant current didactic curriculum, or whether it can be added without increasing student curricular hours.

Gross Anatomy

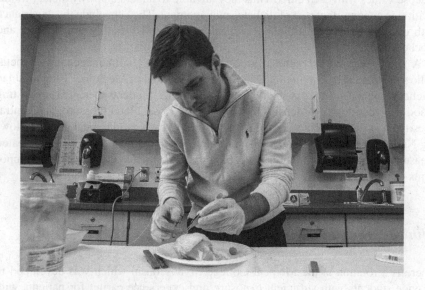

Gross anatomy is one of the prime examples of laboratory teaching, although it has changed with the advent of computer simulation and prosected models as many medical schools have moved away from cadaver-based dissection. This specific example pertains to a small exercise within the overall gross anatomy course. At our institution, clinicians, primarily surgeons, participate in the gross anatomy lab in order to focus the students on why learning anatomy is important. Several times during the semester, these clinicians come to the anatomy lab to demonstrate procedures on the cadavers—central line insertion, chest tube insertion, tracheostomy, laparoscopic cholecystectomy, and placement of orthopedic traction pins. The students are given a handout before each session that describes both the technical details of the procedure and the relevant anatomy. Clinicians teach the procedure at the "bedside" of each cadaver, allowing interested students to perform the procedure. Clearly, the first-year students will not become proficient in chest tube placement after this exercise. However, they have a better understanding of why time spent learning anatomy is important, and they sincerely appreciate the early interaction with clinicians.

Biochemistry/Physiology

A significant percentage of people with diabetes are unaware of their condition. The majority of medical students will treat patients with diabetes in their practice, and many will have the opportunity for initial diagnosis. To highlight some of the management issues facing patients with diabetes and teach about glucose metabolism, first-year students participate in a blood glucose lab in the biochemistry course in our curriculum. Students come to class after an overnight fast, learn how to use lancets to measure their own blood glucose, and take a baseline reading. They then eat breakfast provided for them—either high fiber, high simple sugar, or high fat. Glucose readings are taken throughout the morning, and students compare their glucose values with each other. Thus they are able to understand why dietary modification is an important part of diabetes management. They conclude the experience with discussions led by a diabetic educator, nutritionist, family practitioner, and biochemist.

A similar laboratory centered around the diagnosis and management of metabolic syndrome is held at the Indiana University School of Medicine. The initial lab teaches students how to draw blood from one another. Students then measure fasting blood triglycerides, high-density lipoproteins, glucose, blood pressure, and central obesity on each other. They are then randomized to eat a regular meal or one following National Cholesterol Education Program Step I or II diets. Often with repeated measurements, discussion about physiological, nutritional, and behavioral components of the syndrome ensues.

Clinical Procedures

There is a rotation at the Medical College of Wisconsin which was developed to provide students with sufficient exposure and experience caring for patients with acute life-threatening disease. The rotation includes having the students read chest radiographs with examples of traumatic pathology, placement of chest tubes and performing a cricothyroidotomy on a mannequin, placing skeletal traction devices on one another, and reading computed tomographic scans. All skills are performed with a faculty instructor in a small group setting in the context of case-based scenarios.

The key to this type of lab experience is the integration of didactic discussion with the laboratory and simulation experience. Furthermore, allowing the students to work in small groups makes them active participants in the educational process. Providing students with multiple ways to learn the material increases their enthusiasm as well as their understanding of the concepts. Similar experiences exist in many other places; some may be an entire course or rotation, while others are smaller components of larger rotations that may combine several different learning experiences.

This is clearly not an exhaustive list. Other successful laboratory exercises include performing electrocardiograms during a cardiac physiology unit, measurement of pulmonary function before and after exercise to demonstrate respiratory physiology in action, participating in noninvasive ventilation to learn about various ventilator modes, and others. Orthopedic labs use power tools and clamps purchased at the hardware store, and porous hard foam to simulate bones. Pigs feet and hooks mounted on wooden boards work well for basic suturing and knot tying skills.

Developing Goals and Objectives for Laboratory Teaching

It is tempting to jump on the laboratory exercises bandwagon based on enthusiastic student response and belief in a good idea. BEWARE—laboratory exercises are meant to be part of an educational program, and must have clear goals, objectives, and outcomes assessment. Without these, they might be fun, but may not result in improved knowledge or skill, and will certainly require precious faculty time. The following mnemonic is helpful in constructing objectives.

SMART Objectives (Features of Objectives)

1. Specific
2. Measurable
3. Achievable
4. Realistic (or results oriented)
5. Timeframe

Goals and objectives for laboratory teaching will depend on the experience level of the student and where the laboratory is placed in the curriculum. They will also depend on whether the laboratory exercise is designed to supplant or enhance current curriculum.

A couple of examples illustrate the range of possible objectives. In the case where the exercise is supplanting didactic, teacher-based learning, existing goals and objectives will likely need to be covered. In the case where the exercise is enhancing current curriculum, existing goals and objectives should be modified or additional ones developed. Several broad goals are possible, including skill acquisition, integration of basic science and clinical concepts, and early introduction of clinical faculty to medical students.

If the goal is skill acquisition, the objective would be demonstration of technical competence or proficiency. This is exemplified in the clinical procedures rotation above; the students are expected to demonstrate correct performance of a cricothyroidotomy and chest tube placement on a mannequin. For the clinician involvement in gross anatomy described above, the two goals do not relate to skill acquisition despite the fact that the laboratory experience is skill-centered. The goals of the lab are recognition of the importance of anatomy and early exposure of first-year medical students to practicing clinicians; the objectives are naming important anatomic structures relevant to each skill and individual conversations between students and clinicians. Similarly, the goal of the glucose lab is to understand the importance of diet and nutrition in the management of diabetes, with the objective of demonstrating differences in blood glucose after ingestion of different meals.

Assessment of Laboratory Teaching Exercises

It is important to consider assessment of student learning, or performance, as a well defined aspect of the educational experience. Both formative and summative assessment strategies may be applied to the laboratory setting. Assessment should be linked to the goals, objectives, and instructional methods in a manner that makes intuitive sense. If the objective is to identify the anatomic structures of the hand, then the assessment tool should include some form of labeling activity. For labs designed to teach skill acquisition, the appropriate method of assessment should be demonstration of the skill or a formal Objective Structured Assessment of Clinical Skill (OSCE) or Objective Structured Assessment of Technical Skill (OSATS). If the laboratory exercise is designed to enhance knowledge acquisition, a traditional multiple choice question examination is sufficient. To assess deeper understanding and decision making, an OSCE can provide excellent formative and summative assessment information. For laboratory exercises that are designed to influence perceptions, surveys or questionnaires are best (Table 9.1).

How to Set-Up a Lab Exercise

Laboratory set-up consists of two parts—instructor preparation and space/equipment considerations. Although space and equipment are clearly important, it is far more likely that instructor preparation will not get enough attention. Many teachers, comfortable with teacher-centered didactic instruction, will either not feel the need or not know how to do any preparatory work for a student-centered laboratory exercise. Inexperienced leaders of these exercises often make the assumption that facilitating student-centered learning is something that anyone who has been in an instructor/teaching role can do. The instructors or facilitators should receive a copy of the goals and objectives for the laboratory exercise, as well as the assessment tool, before the lab. They should be familiar with the conduct of the lab, and for a skills lab should be able to perform the skill with the available equipment. The students do not want to hear "well, this isn't really the way I do it" or "I'm really not sure why they are having you do it this way."

Table 9.1 Matching of goals/objectives with assessment methods for lab exercises

Objective	Assessment method
Skill acquisition	Skill demonstration
	OSCE
	OSATS
Knowledge acquisition	Multiple choice examination
Decision making/critical thinking	OSCE
Influence or determine perception or opinion	Survey
	Questionnaire

Instructors may need an introduction or refresher on "how to teach" active learning. A part of this introduction may need to address biases against active learning:

1. It lessens overall quality—the students could be listening to me lecture rather than doing this silly grade-school exercise.
2. Teaching does not occur unless knowledge is transferred from one individual to another.
3. An instructor's job requires that all material must be covered in the allotted time.

Specific behaviors that promote success in an active learning environment include:

1. Moving around the room and interacting with multiple students.
2. Asking directed or targeted, open-ended questions of specific students.
3. Asking students to reflect on what they have found, what it means, why it happens/happened.
4. Ensure that all students have a chance to participate.

Student preparation is also key. One of the tenets of active learning is that not all learning occurs within the classroom setting. The students should receive any necessary background material prior to the lab exercise, along with a copy of the goals and objectives of the exercise.

Space and equipment considerations and constraints may guide the lab design, although some may be lucky enough to be without constraints. Labs with a single user group require a larger space and less equipment; those with multiple smaller groups can make use of several smaller areas but require more equipment and most often more instructors or facilitators. Grounded electrical outlets with power from either ceiling or floor, special plumbing filters for biohazard material, sinks, freezers, work tables, cabinet space, and protective gear for learners are all additional considerations. Demonstration videos are a nice alternative to live demonstration, particularly when expensive materials are needed; this requires specific AV and computer equipment. However, the quality and availability of handheld video recorders, intra-operative audio-visual equipment, and live streaming of video have expanded the possibilities of video demonstrations greatly.

Consumable supplies can be ordered, but can often be recycled from various places in the hospital. We work with our operating room and supply distribution center to appropriate all usable outdated or expired supplies. This helps keep lab costs down, always important but even more so if the lab is an addition to existing curriculum rather than a replacement. Other ways to reduce costs include collaboration between groups to use all parts of a cadaver and homemade simulators rather than commercially available ones. Wooden slats, plastic wrap, foam and foam tape make a reasonable "simulator" for teaching chest tube placement for a much lower cost than commercially available simulators. Additional options for lowering cost include sharing more expensive resources across several rotations.

Conducting the Lab

Now the fun begins! It is at this point that the focus switches from the teacher to the student and true student-centered, active learning occurs. Make the students commit to an answer prior to performing the exercise or lab—they will retain the information discovered during the lab much better when forced to think through the problem and verbalize the answer beforehand. If possible, encourage the students to work in small groups where peer-to-peer learning can occur; however, ensure that groups are not dominated by a single student. It is frequently helpful to assign students to these small workgroups beforehand.

For skills or procedures, an initial demonstration is imperative. Following the demonstration, some students will want to jump right in and others will want to observe a few more. To a point, this is fine, and likely reflects different learning styles. The instructor's job is to ensure that each student gets enough opportunity to learn and practice. If a student is having difficulty, break the skill down into component tasks and demonstrate each one, having the student practice with immediate feedback.

A potential downside of a student-centered learning environment is that the environment will not stimulate the students to discover or learn the particular point envisioned by the instructor. Under these circumstances you should re-evaluate the exercise and improve the preparation. It is important to clearly delineate the objectives and assess how they will be met. However, problems may also be specific to a particular group of students, so don't change things too quickly. An attentive instructor can easily overcome gaps in achievement of lab objectives. At the conclusion of the lab, the instructor should summarize to ensure that the key points have been made and all of the goals and objectives met. A short summation speech is one way to do this, although it can also be done by eliciting responses from the students and supplementing anything that is missed.

After the Lab

Similar to lab set-up, there are two aspects to consider after the lab is finished. First, the assessment must be complete—often an evaluation is worthwhile even if an MCQ exam or skills demonstration has been the primary method to assess the learner. Prepare good session evaluation forms to get feedback from both students

Table 9.2 Potential pitfalls in laboratory settings

Pitfall	Undesirable outcome
Lack of goals and/or objectives	Waste of faculty time
	No learning occurs
Unprepared or uncomfortable instructors	Disinterested students
	No learning occurs
	Instructor attrition
Learning objective not covered	No learning occurs
No assessment strategy	Inability to judge success of experience
	Unclear if learning occurs

and the instructor. This forethought can be a tremendous help to improve future labs. Furthermore, these evaluations have importance in documenting academic scholarship for the instructors, thereby providing more incentive for faculty participation.

Supplies should be inventoried, and may need to be reordered prior to the next lab. Cleaning, maintenance, and ongoing evaluation of nonconsumable supplies are all necessary to determine whether capital expenditure is required for new equipment.

Pitfalls

The primary result of an unsuccessful laboratory exercise—whatever the reason for lack of success—is that the students will not learn what is intended. Almost all pitfalls are avoidable with a little preparation; it would be a shame to have the work invested in an active learning exercise not result in excited and accomplished learners (Table 9.2).

Summary

There are many opportunities to incorporate these exercises into medical education. With a little preparation, the change in focus from teacher-focused lecturing to student-centered active learning in a laboratory setting can benefit both.

For Further Reading

Fitzpatrick CM, Kolesari GL, Brasel KJ (2003) Surgical origins: new teaching modalities integrating clinical and basic science years-a role for residents as active teachers. Surgery 133(4):353–355

Glasgow SC, Tiemann D, Frisella MM et al (2006) Laparoscopy as an educational and recruiting tool. Am J Surg 191:542–544

Graffam B (2007) Active learning in medical education: strategies for beginning implementation. Med Teach 29:38–42

Gupta S, Westfall TC, Lechner AJ, Knuepfer MM (2005) Teaching principles of cardiovascular function in a medical student laboratory. Adv Physiol Educ 29:118–127

Kolb D (1984) Experiential learning: experience as the source of learning and development. Prentice Hall, Englewood Cliffs

Martin BJ, Watkins JB, Ramsey JW (1998) Venipuncture in the medical physiology laboratory. Adv Physiol Educ 19:S62–S67

Martin B, Watkins JB, Ramsey JW (2004) Evaluating metabolic syndrome in a medical physiology laboratory. Adv Physiol Educ 28:195–198

Michael J (2006) Where's the evidence that active learning works? Adv Physiol Educ 30(4):159–167

Modell HI, Michael JA, Damson T, Horwitz B (2004) Enhancing active learning in the student laboratory. Adv Physiol Educ 28:107–111

Reiter SA, McGill C, Lawrence SL, Twining SS (2000) Blood glucose laboratory for first-year medical students: an interdisciplinary model for nutrition focused diabetes management. J Am Dietetic Assoc 100:570–572

University of Buffalo, National Center for Case Study, Teaching in Science. http://ublib.buffalo.edu/libraries/projects/cases. Accessed 1 Mar 2014

University of Medicine and Dentistry of New Jersey, Center for Teaching Excellence. http://cte.umdnj.edu/active_learning. Accessed 1 Mar 2014

White J, Paslawski T, Kearney R (2013) 'Discovery Learning': an account of rapid curriculum change in response to accreditation. Med Teach 35:e1319–e1326

Chapter 10
Teaching with Technological Tools

David A. Cook

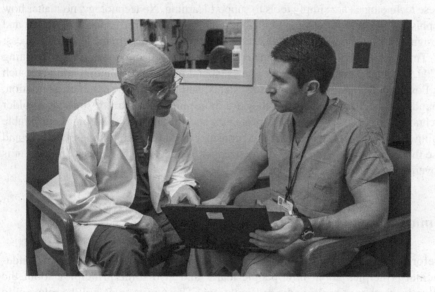

Abstract Computer-based instructional tools are just the latest in a long line of educational technologies that probably started when someone picked up a piece of cinder and wrote on a cave wall. It is common to become fascinated – or infatuated – with new technologies, but it is important to remember that these technologies are simply tools to support learning. No technology, no matter how sophisticated, will supplant a skilled teacher, effective instructional methods and designs, or – most importantly – the central role of the student in the learning process. This chapter

D.A. Cook, M.D., MHPE (✉)
Division of General Internal Medicine, Mayo Clinic College of Medicine,
200 First St. SW, Rochester, MN 55905, USA
e-mail: cook.david33@mayo.edu

K.N. Huggett and W.B. Jeffries (eds.), *An Introduction to Medical Teaching*,
DOI 10.1007/978-94-017-9066-6_10, © Springer Science+Business Media Dordrecht 2014

will discuss how tools such as computer-based tutorials, virtual patients, just-in-time learning, presentation software, audience response systems, and videos can be used to effectively enhance learning.

Introduction

The first use of educational technology probably occurred when someone picked up a stick and drew in the sand, or when someone picked up a piece of cinder and wrote on a cave wall. Chalk, papyrus, paintings, printed books, chalkboards, and more recently photographs, overhead projectors, televisions, and computers all represent technological advances that can used for educational purposes. It is common to become fascinated – or infatuated – with new technologies, but it is important to remember that these technologies are simply tools to support learning. No technology, no matter how sophisticated, will supplant a skilled teacher, effective instructional methods and designs, or – most importantly – the central role of the student in the learning process.

This chapter will focus on newer technologies – computer-assisted learning (CAL), virtual patients, computer games, social media, presentation software such as PowerPoint™, audience response systems, and multimedia (graphics, animation, sound and video) – not because they are more important than or superior to older technologies, but simply because they are new and educators must become comfortable using them. However, teachers should consider all of the technologies available and use those methods that best serve the needs of the learner. The use of simulation is covered in another chapter in this book.

Fundamental Principles

Before discussing any specific technologies it is worth reviewing a few fundamental principles about how people learn, and also some principles about the effective design of multimedia presentations. These principles will be relevant to all of the educational technologies subsequently discussed, and are summarized in Tables 10.1 and 10.2.

Core Principles of Instructional Design

As in all instruction, the use of educational technology should focus on helping learners effectively construct new knowledge rather than trying to effectively transmit information. Learning is more than accumulation of information, but rather involves organizing, reorganizing, and linking new information and experiences with prior knowledge and past experience. This process, known as elaboration, constitutes the core of all learning. Educational technologies will be

Table 10.1 Principles of effective multimedia learning

Principle	Learning is enhanced when…
Multimedia principle	Both words and graphics (pictorial information) are used
Modality principle and redundancy principle	Descriptions of graphics are spoken rather than appearing as on-screen text, but concurrent written and spoken text are avoided
Contiguity principle	Related information (graphics and accompanying explanation; instructions; feedback) is placed close together (on the same page, and close together on page)
Coherence principle	Only necessary information (graphics, words, sound) is presented
Personalization principle	A conversational tone is used
Learner pacing principle	Learners can control the pace of the course
Guided discovery principle	Structure (content selection, sequencing, and interpretation) is present for novice learners
Worked example principle	Some (but not all) practice problems are replaced with worked examples
Expertise-reversal effect	Structure and worked examples are provided for novice learners, while advanced learners receive less structure and unsolved problems

See Clark and Mayer (2007) for details and additional principles of multimedia learning

Table 10.2 General tips when using educational technologies

Consider the need for educational technology: Are simpler technologies or traditional instructional methods adequate? Is this the *best* technology to meet the needs of this group/content/context?

Spend less time/energy/money on bells and whistles, and more time planning for effective learner interaction

Consider how you will stimulate active learning

  Structure learning around a problem (e.g., patient case)

  Activate prior knowledge, demonstrate, allow opportunity for application and integration

Follow principles of effective multimedia learning

Provide time for learning; set deadlines

Practice or pilot the course before implementation

most effective inasmuch as they encourage learners to construct robust, meaningful knowledge structures.

In considering how to accomplish this, Merrill (2002) reviewed the literature looking for common themes among various educational theories and models, and distilled five "first principles of instructional design." First and foremost, all instruction should be situated in the context of real life *problems*. This is not synonymous with problem-based learning per se, but rather implies that patient cases (or other relevant problems) should figure centrally in all instruction. The second principle is *activation* – "learning is promoted when relevant previous experience is activated." Activation means that prior knowledge (including formal instruction and lived experiences) is brought to the forefront of working memory, where it can be integrated with new experiences and information. The third principle is *demonstration* – "learning is promoted when the instruction demonstrates what is to be learned, rather than merely telling information about what is to be learned." Next comes *application* – "learning is promoted when learners are required to use new knowledge or skills to solve problems." Guidance and coaching should be provided initially, and then be gradually withdrawn such that in the end learners can solve problems independently. Finally, *integration* – "learning is promoted when learners are encouraged to integrate (transfer) the new knowledge or skill into their everyday lives."

Designing Effective Multimedia

Based on decades of empiric research, Mayer (see Clark and Mayer 2007) has formulated several principles of effective multimedia learning (Table 10.1). These principles are relevant to computer-assisted instruction, PowerPoint™ presentations, and other uses of audio and video in instruction.

Multimedia Principle: People Learn More from Graphics and Words than from Words Alone

A picture is worth a 1,000 words, and it comes as no surprise that graphics, photographs, animations, and short video clips can greatly enhance learning. Graphics help learners construct effective mental representations. While irrelevant graphics actually detract from learning (see below), relevant graphics can be used to illustrate examples (and non-examples) of an object, to provide a topic overview or organization scheme, to demonstrate steps in a procedure or process, or to illuminate complex relationships among content, concepts, or time or space.

Modality Principle: When There Are Graphics, Present Words as Speech Rather than Onscreen Text

New information can reach working memory through separate visual and auditory pathways. Learning is maximized when both pathways are optimally used. For example, a graphic accompanied by spoken explanation (both pathways used) will be more effective than the same graphic accompanied by onscreen text (vision-only). Paradoxically, when identical information reaches working memory simultaneously via both vision and hearing (such as when a presenter reads their PowerPoint™ slides verbatim) it can actually impair, rather then enhance, learning. Thus, the modality principle encourages teachers to maximize mental capacities by using both visual and phonetic information, while avoiding redundancy (presenting identical text onscreen and as speech).

Contiguity Principle: Related Information Should Be Placed Close Together

It is common to include an explanatory legend at the bottom of a figure. However, this physical separation of information wastes mental energy that could be better spent on learning. It is far more effective to place the explanatory text within the figure itself. This helps learners appreciate relationships (=build meaningful knowledge), and it minimizes the cognitive effort spent going back and forth between a figure and the accompanying text. The same principle applies to non-graphical elements, such as putting the directions for an exercise on the same page as the exercise itself, or presenting the question and the answer/feedback together when providing formative feedback on an online test.

Coherence Principle: Avoid the Extraneous (Less Is More)

Interesting but irrelevant details detract from learning. This includes sounds, graphics, or unnecessary words. Teachers often add cartoons or photos to presentations for aesthetic value (to "spice up" a lecture), but such decorative graphics can actually impede learning rather than enhance it. The same applies to extraneous sounds, interesting but irrelevant stories, unnecessarily detailed descriptions, and most animations. Not only does extraneous information tax cognitive capacities, it can also *distract* the learner from more relevant material, *disrupt* the learner from building appropriate mental links, and *seduce* learning by activating inappropriate prior knowledge which leads to flawed knowledge structures. The purpose of words, graphics, and multimedia in instruction is to help learners construct mental representations. If they do not serve this purpose, they should probably be removed. As John Dewey once stated, "When things have to be made interesting it is because interest itself is wanting. The thing, the object is no more interesting than it was before." (Dewey 1913, pp. 11–12) Bottom line: if it doesn't facilitate learning, leave it out.

Guided Discovery Principle, Worked Example Principle, and Expertise Reversal Effect

Many educators have advocated unstructured learning environments, claiming that freeing learners from the tethers of rigid instruction will enhance learning. However, abundant research suggests that this is not the case – at least, not all the time. The guided discovery principle states that learning is enhanced when information is presented in a planned sequence and when learners are assisted in their interpretation of this information – in short, when learners are guided in the learning process. This guidance need not be excessive. In fact, too much guidance diminishes the need for learners to think deeply about new information and weakens the resultant knowledge structures. The worked example principle is similar, namely that learning is enhanced when some practice problems are replaced with worked examples.

However, as learners advance they require progressively less guidance and become increasingly independent in solving problems. This transition from supported to independent learning and problem solving has been labeled the **expertise reversal effect**. What works for novices will not work for more advanced learners, and what works for advanced learners won't work for novices. Learners should initially be provided guidance and worked examples, and progress to independence.

Educational Technologies as "Mindtools"

Jonassen (2000) has suggested that students should learn *with* computers rather than *from* computers. By this he means that instead of sitting in front of a computer tutorial, students should use computer-based tools such as word processing, spreadsheet, and database programs; programs to generate semantic maps; and online discussion as "Mindtools" to facilitate knowledge elaboration. Other educators have assigned learners to produce PowerPoint™ presentations, web pages, or video clips related to the topic of study. This paradigm – using computers and other technologies as knowledge organization tools, rather than tools for the transmission of knowledge – merits consideration and further research.

Faculty Training

A critical, but often overlooked, issue in the use of educational technologies is faculty training. Training needs include the technical and instructional skills (they are different!) required to develop an effective educational object such as a CAL module, PowerPoint™ presentation, or video clip, and the skills to integrate these objects effectively into a course. This chapter provides an introduction for faculty that focuses on the instructional aspects.

Is There a "Net Generation"?

Some authors have proposed that people born after the advent of digital technologies have a natural aptitude for using these technologies, while those born earlier will never catch up. A corollary to this argument is that those in the younger "Net Generation" have an inherent desire and expectation to use these technologies in all phases of life, including learning. The implication is that educators and schools must deliberately develop and use these technologies in their teaching practice, even if such use requires acquiring new infrastructure and skills, and hiring new specialists with expertise in technology-enhanced instructional design.

However, evidence suggests these "generations" are a myth – at least insofar as they have relevance to education (Jones and Shao 2011). Studies show little difference among age cohorts in the use of e-mail, mobile devices, and social media such as Facebook. More importantly, surveys suggest that younger students don't necessarily prefer to learn using these new technologies, and in some cases would prefer to have more face-to-face time with instructors. The bottom line is that teachers and administrators should feel empowered, but not obligated, to use and support these new technologies.

Computer-Assisted Learning

We will now discuss a number of specific educational technologies, beginning with CAL. CAL in all forms requires a paradigm shift for the teacher. Direct interaction with the learner is greatly reduced or eliminated altogether. However, the teacher continues to interact indirectly by virtue of the course/website design and the instructional methods selected.

There is nothing magical about CAL that makes it inherently better than other forms of instruction (such as face-to-face lectures or small groups). Decades of research have failed to detect any consistent advantage once changes in the instructional design/method are accounted for. Hence, educators should not jump to CAL as a solution for all instructional problems. Indeed, it will often be an inferior choice. Sometimes traditional methods will be more effective. However, blended learning, which uses creative combinations of CAL and traditional methods, is increasingly recognized as the ideal solution for many situations. Among other blended approaches, CAL can facilitate a "**flipped classroom**," (see Chap. 4) in which students complete the bulk of their studying and homework before the face-to-face class session. Since students arrive having already mastered the fundamentals, teachers can use precious face-to-face time for activities that reinforce and extend learning and application. The concept of pre-learning certainly isn't new, but CAL enables novel pre-class approaches such as short video lectures, online discussion, and online assessment.

CAL comes in many flavors or configurations, including tutorials, online communities, virtual patients, performance support, online resources, and portfolios. Each of these will be discussed in turn.

Computer-Based Tutorials

What It Is

Computer-based tutorials are similar to face-to-face lectures. They consist of structured information, often enhanced by multimedia and interactivity. Such tutorials are often Web-based, although they can also be implemented on specific computers or using digital media.

When to Use

Computer-based (and in particular Web-based) tutorials have advantages such as flexibility in the physical location or timing of participation; the presentation of a consistent and easily updated message; learner self-pacing; facilitation of assessment and documentation; and a number of novel instructional methods that are difficult to implement in other modalities. However, there are also a number of disadvantages, including difficulty in adapting to individual needs; social isolation; development and maintenance costs; and technical problems. Computer-based tutorials will be most useful when learners are separated in time or space (such as conflicting schedules or rotations at different sites).

How to Use

When planning a CAL tutorial, it is important to do your homework. The initial development costs are likely to be great (perhaps much more than you anticipate), and this and other disadvantages should be balanced against potential advantages. Be sure that you have adequate technical support at your institution. Consider who will be doing the programming and who will provide technical support when problems arise. If commercial software meeting your needs is available, it may be cheaper to purchase this rather than develop a new program in-house. Proprietary learning management systems such as Blackboard or free, open-source systems such as Moodle can be helpful in organizing your course.

When developing the course itself, pay attention to the design principles noted above. In particular, remember that the goal of instruction is mental activity on the part of the learner – elaboration of information and construction of new knowledge. Physical activity (such as clicking the mouse) does not guarantee mental activity; direct your design to facilitate mental activity. Opportunities for self assessment and feedback, reflection, and interaction with other learners can facilitate this. Also, well designed interactive components can help. However, keep in mind the coherence principle – if it does not add to learning leave it out. Clark and Mayer (2007) provide additional considerations in thorough detail.

Also pay close attention to the website design. In addition to Mayer's principles, Web pages should be organized for consistency and clarity. Use the same basic layout from one page to the next within your course. Create a visual hierarchy to focus attention, and chunk related information together. Make it clear at all times, "What can I do on this screen, and where do I need to go next?"

Before implementation, pilot the website in terms of both functionality and appearance. Make the website readily accessible to learners. Secure commitment from all stakeholders – not just from the administration, but also from faculty and learners. Don't forget to provide time for learning. There is temptation to tack a Web-based course onto an already full schedule. CAL permits flexible scheduling, but does not prolong the hours of the day. Table 10.3 summarizes these recommendations.

Table 10.3 Tips for computer-based tutorials

Use commercial software if it meets your needs
Get buy-in from administration, faculty, and students
Distinguish physical and mental activity: clicking mouse/=learning; try to stimulate mental activity
Make site accessible and user-friendly

Something New: MOOCs

In the past few years, massive open online courses (MOOCs) have emerged as a new model for distance learning. These online courses are massive (enrolling thousands or even hundreds of thousands of students) and open (anyone can enroll free of charge). Dropout rates are high – often upwards of 90 % – but hundreds or thousands of people still complete the course, and thousands more obtain initial exposure to the topic (and the professor and school). Computers can potentially track all course activity – even typing speed and pausing or speeding up a video – and use this information for assessment (e.g., to verify understanding), evaluation (to identify areas for course improvement), and personalization (to adapt to individual needs). While enrollment is free, participants typically pay for assessment activities and for a certificate of completion. At the time of writing, MOOCs are so new that it is impossible to predict what will happen – but as a "disruptive technology" they deserve attention.

Online Communities: Blogs, Wikis, and Discussion Boards

What It Is

Internet-mediated communication has facilitated the development of so-called online learning communities. In the virtual equivalent of a face-to-face small group discussion, learners can interact to share experiences and information and learn collaboratively. As with face-to-face small groups, online learner interaction serves both a social function and as a stimulus to active learning.

Much online communication is asynchronous – i.e., there is a delay between sending a message and receiving the response. Tools for asynchronous communication include e-mail, unthreaded and threaded discussion boards, blogs, and wikis. Synchronous communication is real-time, and is mediated through Internet audio or video chat (e.g., Skype, Google Hangouts, and Apple Facetime) and instant messaging. Unthreaded discussions are typically arranged chronologically (i.e., with most recent posts at the bottom or top). Threaded discussions are organized in a hierarchical or topic fashion, with each response to a message appearing immediately after that message. Blogs (short for web logs) consist of dated posts organized in reverse chronological order; usually only one person (the author) contributes to the posts, although there is often a provision for visitors to comment. Wikis, from the Hawaiian word for quick, allow all users to contribute to revisions of the same document or web page. A growing number of free and paid Internet resources can support these and other online collaborative activities.

When to Use

The advantages and disadvantages of online communities compared to face-to-face small groups are similar to those described above for tutorials. They will be most useful when learners are unable to meet together face-to-face (in fact, it is probably preferable for learners to meet in person when possible). One might choose threaded discussion when the emphasis is organization of communication around specific themes or topics; blogs when the goal is documentation of personal impressions, such as e-portfolios (discussed in greater detail later on) or a journal; and wikis when the objective is a collaboratively developed final product.

Social media tools can also play an important role in building online learning communities. Students have used social media (e.g., Facebook) to form online study groups, and instructors have used it both for social purposes (team building) and to replace tools designed for instruction (discussion boards, white boards, etc.). One problem is that the functions that promote social interactions are often not ideal for instructional activities. For example, users have encountered challenges in following long conversations, limitations on accepted file formats, and distractions that encourage socializing rather than studying. Yet, since such tools are widely accessible and essentially free, there may be pragmatic reasons to use them even if the interface is not ideal.

How to Use

After deciding to develop an online learning community and selecting the appropriate configuration, the next step is to identify or train a qualified facilitator. Effective online small-group facilitation requires a unique skill set. The "e-moderator" must ask questions, challenge points of view, provide summaries and synthesis, redirect when a discussion goes astray, promote active participation from all group members, and encourage a healthy social environment. At the same time, the facilitator must remain a "guide on the side" and ensure that the learning evolves from group collaboration.

Online learning communities seem to work best when some degree of structure is provided. The facilitator will typically pose a question or specific task to the members of the group. For example, a problem-based learning task might give a group an unstructured case and ask members to analyze the case (see Chap. 4), identify problems, and come up with a solution. Case analysis is similar but emphasizes the identification of root causes of the problem rather than solutions, often considering multiple different paradigms or perspectives. Critical incident discussions ask students to identify a formative experience (such as an influential positive role model, or an error made in patient care) and identify salient details of this incident. Groups then identify common themes among their experiences.

It is often helpful to assign students to work in groups of two to five to ensure that everyone has an opportunity to participate. There are various permutations on this theme, such as breaking apart and reorganizing groups halfway through an assignment, encouraging participants to work as individuals initially and then collaborate for the final product, or begin as a group and then submit a final product written alone. Wikis allow groups to work collaboratively on a single final product. Firm deadlines should be fixed well in advance (on or before the first day of the course, if possible). Interim deadlines are useful as well.

It is often appropriate for the facilitator to post resources such as journal articles and book chapters (provided copyright law is taken into account), written introductions or summaries, slide presentations, or links to external websites. However, these should not supplant the collaborative group learning process.

Two serious threats to online communities are inflammatory communications between group members and silence. The first problem ("flaming") can lead to a loss of mutual trust and disintegration of the collaborative environment. Those involved in heated discussions should be redirected by the facilitator, and if this proves unsuccessful they may need to be excluded from participation. "Lurkers" read messages but do not post responses. Not only are such individuals less likely to learn deeply, but by failing to contribute they negatively affect the experience for all. After detecting lurking, facilitators should first try encouraging participation from all participants generally. If this is unsuccessful they may need to resort to one-on-one communication with the individual student.

Learners should be taught the rules of "netiquette" that govern online communication. First and foremost be polite. Learners should carefully proofread messages before posting and consider whether their words could be misinterpreted. Typos can be confusing, and small errors in spelling and punctuation can completely change the meaning of a sentence or paragraph. Writing in ALL CAPS is considered yelling and should be avoided. Empty messages such as "I agree" should be shunned in favor of more informative comments (for example, explaining *why* the individual agreed). Participants should carefully read what has been previously posted to avoid repeating comments. Humor should be employed with great caution: without voice inflection and physical gestures it is easy for messages to be misinterpreted. Finally, to the extent possible it is usually preferable that all communication in the community be done in a common forum (such as the discussion thread), so that everyone can learn together. The one exception is when personal feedback from instructor to student might be inappropriate for a group setting (such as from the facilitator to someone who is flaming or lurking). Table 10.4 summarizes tips for online communities.

Table 10.4 Tips for developing online learning communities

Choose a configuration appropriate to learning goals: email, threaded discussion, blog, wiki
Train the facilitator
Assign tasks that promote meaningful collaboration and learning
Develop the social aspects of the group
Beware of lurkers and flaming
Judiciously incorporate online resources such as websites, documents, multimedia, and slide presentations
Teach "netiquette": participate, be polite (proofread messages, review for alternate interpretations, no personal attacks), avoid all capital letters, no empty messages

Something New: Virtual Worlds

Virtual Worlds such as Second Life allow users to "live in" a simulated environment and interact via avatars, which are graphical representations of real people (i.e., other users and instructors). As with most new technologies, educators have creatively used Second Life for teaching purposes. Students (or rather, their avatars) can attend virtual lectures and workshops; interact in problem-based learning discussions, team building activities, and collaborative projects; and manage virtual patients. Research on virtual worlds is thus far limited to descriptive studies, and it remains unclear how this technology will compare with other technologies that promote online collaboration.

Virtual Patients

What It Is

A virtual patient is "a specific type of computer-based program that simulates real-life clinical scenarios; learners emulate the roles of health care providers to obtain a history, conduct a physical exam, and make diagnostic and therapeutic decisions" (AAMC Report 2007). The defining feature (and limitation) is the attempt to mimic reality on a computer screen. Virtual patients can range from patient cases that develop linearly with occasional prompts for the learner to make decisions or request additional information, to complex simulations that branch in response to learner questions and actions.

When to Use

The evidence base regarding virtual patients is limited (see Cook and Triola 2009), and most recommendations are based either on extrapolation from other forms of CAL or on conjecture and expert opinion. The most appropriate role of virtual patients appears to be the development of clinical reasoning. Lectures and CAL tutorials are probably superior for the development of core knowledge, and standardized patients or real patients are superior for the development of history taking, examination, and counseling skills. However, a growing body of evidence suggests that there are no generic problem solving skills in medicine (or any other subject), but rather that problem solving skills (such as diagnostic reasoning or selection among management options – collectively termed clinical reasoning) involve a large amount of pattern recognition. Hence, the development of clinical reasoning requires a large number of patterns, which derives from seeing lots of patients. If real-life experience is insufficient, supplementing the mental case library with simulated experiences may help. Virtual patients provide an efficient way to provide such experiences.

How to Use

The key consideration in teaching with virtual patients involves the selection, sequencing, and implementation of cases. Ideally, cases on a given topic would start off relatively simple (and perhaps with some guidance in decision-making) and progress to more challenging cases with greater complexity and less guidance. Looking to facilitate elaboration (which George Bordage (1994) has termed "the key to successful diagnostic thinking"), teachers might encourage learners to explicitly contrast two or more cases, to justify the elements of history, exam, and laboratory testing they select, to rank diagnoses in the order of probability, to explain how their choices might change with a slight variation in the clinical scenario, or to identify the evidence in favor of their management strategy. Feedback might consist of an expert's approach to the same case, an index of concordance with accepted guidelines, or measures of cost or time efficiency.

Regarding the design and implementation of virtual patients, technological sophistication does not equate with better learning. Much attention is paid to the fidelity or realism of the virtual patient. However, these concerns are likely ill-founded. Not only is high fidelity expensive, but there is some evidence to suggest that it can paradoxically impede rather than enhance learning. Likewise, while intuition suggests that asking learners to type questions into the computer to elicit a history may be most effective, evidence suggests that selecting questions from a preset list of standard questions may be more effective. Finally, many virtual patients require learners to click on specific body organs to examine them. It is unclear whether this activity enhances learning (mental activity) or merely represents physical interactivity.

The development of a good virtual patient library can be difficult. Not only are scenario scripts time-consuming to prepare, but the technology to turn a script into a working virtual patient can be expensive. Efforts such as the MedBiquitous virtual patient standards group and the AAMC's MedEdPortal are working to facilitate the sharing of such resources among institutions. Authoring tools such as OpenLabyrinth, CASUS, and WebSP can help, and commercial products such as DxR Clinician should also be considered.

Even after cases have been developed, there is still the issue of how to integrate these into a curriculum. Some educators have found that working through a virtual case as a group is more effective than working alone, or that virtual patients are most effective as part of a blended learning activity (for example, having a face-to-face group discussion once everyone has completed the case). Additional considerations include: Will cases be mandatory or optional? What is the right balance between virtual patients and real patients? Are learners who have seen real patients with a similar problem able to opt out? How will learners find time to work on cases? What training will teachers need in the use of the software and specific cases, and how will institutional buy-in be achieved?

Just-In-Time Learning (Performance Support)

What It Is

Just-in-time learning involves delivering educational information at critical stages in a clinical encounter (performance support). Information can be "pushed" to the provider (such as automated feedback in response to specific triggers in computerized order entry, feedback linked with electronic prescribing patterns, or CAL packages that tailor their activity and response to individual practice patterns) or "pulled" by the provider (from online searchable knowledge resources). The essence is that the learner (who is often a practicing healthcare professional) can either seek, or be automatically provided with, information relevant to the patient sitting in his or her office. The theoretical educational advantages are at least twofold. First, this is a moment when learners (practitioners) might be particularly receptive to the material, since it (hopefully) will enable them to provide improved patient care. Second, because a knowledge gap has been identified and prior knowledge activated, learners are potentially primed to integrate this new information into their existing knowledge structure.

When to Use

Just-in-time learning is used when learners (providers) are seeing patients. As useful as this sounds, it has limitations. It takes time to read, digest, and assimilate this information in a busy clinical schedule, and learners may resent mandatory pop- ups or unsolicited e-mail reminders if these affect their practice efficiency. Also, just-in-time learning may not substitute for other instructional approaches because the ad hoc, unstructured information may be improperly integrated. For example, a teaching point relevant to one patient may be over-generalized to a population for whom a different rule should apply; or the knowledge structure may be left with gaps not addressed by the performance support system. Thus, performance support – at least at present – is just that: support. It should not replace (at least not completely) other instructional methods.

How to Use

The paucity of evidence makes specific recommendations difficult; however the suggestions for CAL tutorials likely apply. Additional questions to consider include how much information to present, how to organize and structure this information to facilitate meaningful learning, how to motivate learning, and what will trigger the information to appear? Effective instructional methods (which usually take more time) must be balanced against the time constraints of a busy clinical practice. As evidence and experience accumulate, performance support systems will, in coming years, likely become more prevalent and employ more effective instructional designs.

Online resources such as UpToDate and Google™ have become the first line information source for many practitioners. However, the availability of such resources does not guarantee that they will be used, or used effectively. The same pedagogical concerns described above for "pushed" information apply here.

Something New: Mobile Devices

Since the last edition of this book, the use of mobile technologies has skyrocketed. The iPhone had only recently been announced – and the iPad was only a rumor – at that time. These and other mobile devices are now ubiquitous, and perhaps their greatest educational impact has been in facilitating just-in-time learning. These devices allow teachers and learners to quite literally take learning to the patient's bedside. Although educators continue to struggle with screen size limitations and the other challenges noted above, mobile learning has much to offer to medical education.

Portfolios and Online Assessment Tools

What It Is

An important part of teaching is learner assessment, and computers can facilitate this in numerous ways. The administration of online self-assessment and summative tests is now commonplace, and typically allows automated grading and immediate personalized feedback. Education portfolios can include a variety of information and "artifacts" relevant to a student's professional development, similar to an artist's portfolio of completed works. Relevant information might include case reports, patient logs, records (written, audiotaped, or videotaped) of performance, essays, research project reports, and self-reflection narratives. Online tools can simplify such portfolios. Logbooks are a specific type of portfolio used to keep track of procedures performed and patients seen.

When to Use

Online self-assessments are useful as pretests, interim tests, or posttests to help learners identify strengths and knowledge gaps. Formative feedback can itself be a powerful instructional method. Online summative assessments can be used for grading and documentation in addition to providing feedback.

Portfolios are particularly helpful in assessing domains that do not lend themselves to multiple-choice tests, such as attitudes, critical thinking, application of theory to practice, and progress over time. Since students study what will be tested, portfolios provide one way for teachers to emphasize these important elements of training. Reflection itself is an important instructional method that can be facilitated by portfolios. Portfolios will likely see greater use as the limitations of existing assessment tools are increasingly recognized.

How to Use

Specific information on assessing student performance can be found in Chap. 15. Many commercial and open-source tools are available to facilitate online testing.

When considering an online portfolio, the first decision is what type of information you wish students to include. These materials should align with the objectives of the course or curriculum. Students will need clear guidelines about the type of materials to be included and the narrative or explanation to accompany each component. Deadlines are important. Clear grading criteria, aligned with the objectives of the course, will need to be established and shared with the student. Such criteria might assess the organization of materials; the amount of thought and reflection evidenced in discussion; and other criteria specific to the type of material included (such as scores on a multiple choice test, or scientific rigor in a report on a research activity). Faculty development may be needed for both the faculty members who assist the students in developing the portfolio, and also those who assign grades.

Software for the development of online portfolios could be as simple as a blog or a wiki, or the student's personal page in a learning management system, or a software package designed for this purpose. Mobile devices are now used for many portfolio purposes, including patient tracking and procedural logbooks.

Educational Games

What It Is

Educational games are activities with rules and a defined outcome (winning, losing) or other feedback (e.g. points) that facilitate comparisons of performance. Games typically have explicit goals and a compelling storyline, and thus have the potential to engage learners and encourage their continued practice with the objective of improved knowledge and skill acquisition and application. However, the benefits of online educational games in medical education are still largely hypothetical, with only a few descriptions and even fewer comparative studies.

When to Use

Educational games could be used to augment virtually any course. They could be used to introduce a new subject or to reinforce material recently taught. Two potentially important uses include the management of virtual patients (above) and simulation-based procedural training, both of which require multiple repetitions to achieve proficiency in the target skill.

How to Use

Much remains to be learned about the use of games in medical education. Online gaming technology and authoring tools have made game development more accessible and far less expensive than in the past, but sometimes even a technologically simple game may have benefit. More important than the technology is to focus on a defined instructional objective, to follow the general rules above for instructional design, and to implement the evidence that has accrued for games in non-medical education (see bibliography).

Presentation Support Software

What It Is

Computers are routinely used to support oral presentations. In the 25 years since its first release, PowerPoint™ has developed into a powerful and versatile presentation-support tool. Alternatives to PowerPoint include Apple's Keynote, and Prezi. Software (e.g., Captivate™, Articulate™, and Office Mix™) is also available to turn PowerPoint™ presentations into polished Web-based learning modules. Specially designed screens (Smartboard™) can seamlessly integrate whiteboard techniques (the traditional "chalk talk") with a PowerPoint™ presentation.

When to Use

Although PowerPoint™ presentations are ubiquitous today, for many teaching purposes an open discussion or use of a chalkboard or whiteboard may be more effective. Computer support will be most useful for formal presentations, such as scientific reports, or when multimedia (particularly graphics and photographs) will enhance the teaching session. Narration can also be embedded with the slides, allowing the slideset to serve as a stand-alone learning object (i.e., a very low-tech online learning product). However, presentation software is a tool – and as with all technological tools, can be overused.

How to Use

The trick with presentation software is to use the slides to help the audience mentally engage and visualize the things you are talking about, without distracting them with unnecessary animations, text, or clip art. The principles described above for effective multimedia learning apply to presentation software as much as they do to CAL. In particular, the coherence principle applies to the use of presentation software slides. Most notably, slides should be simple. Use no more than five to seven words per line, and no more than five to seven lines per slide. This may not seem like a lot (and you've likely seen this principle violated frequently) but slides should list merely the key points. You, the teacher, will then elaborate on these points – but if you put full sentences or excessive information, the audience will begin to read your slides (a violation of the redundancy principle). If you must add a direct quote, put only a short excerpt on the slide.

Consistency is a virtue. Using the same fonts, font size, color scheme, and transitions, and even similar clip art styles, will enhance learning by minimizing distraction. In PowerPoint the slide master (View → Master → Slide master) allows you to control default settings for the entire slide show. Never use a font smaller than 28-point. Avoid nonstandard fonts (fancy fonts are both harder to read and also may not be available on a different computer). Colors should contrast, but avoid garish combinations such as green on red. Dark text on light backgrounds is easiest to read. In addition, a light background lends itself to writing on the slide using a SmartBoard™. Each slide design (more below) comes with a palette of colors for text, title, accents, hyperlinks, etc.; try to stick with this palette rather than using other arbitrary colors. Finally, just because presentation software offers lots of options for fancy transitions and animations does not mean you need to use them. In fact, simpler slide shows – with "boring" standard transitions – are usually more effective. Presentation software allows the use of multimedia including clipart, photographs, charts and diagrams, tables, sound, video, and hyperlinks to Internet sites. All of these are useful when used appropriately, but as with everything else can be overdone. Use them only when they truly enhance the presentation.

Presentations often take longer than you think; plan at least 1 min per slide, and time your presentation before presenting. Instead of reading slides verbatim, put only the key points on your slides and then elaborate on these as you talk. Face the audience (not your slides) when presenting. If you are using a video clip be sure to try it out on the computer system you will be using – you may find the clip does not run on a different computer or project well using a different projector. The *speaker notes* (typing text below the slide that is not visible to the audience) can be invaluable both for organizing your thoughts, and also for when you come back to give the presentation again at a later date. Table 10.5 summarizes these and other tips.

Table 10.5 Tips for using presentation software

Spend more time on the content and organization than on designing your slides
Plan for interaction with the audience
Follow the Coherence Principle:
Just the essentials on slides (you'll fill in details verbally)
Simplicity and consistency (use slide master and color scheme)
Bullet points: 5–7 words per line, 7 lines per slide
Large, simple fonts (no less than 28-point font)
Colors: contrasting and vibrant but not garish
Minimize transitions, animations, sound, and other effects
Use clip art, pictures, sound, video, tables, and hyperlinks to support learning (not decoration)
When presenting
If using video: test in advance on presentation computer
Practice and get feedback; time your presentation
Don't read slides, and don't read *to* slides

Lecture Audience Engagement Support

What It Is

Commercially available audience response systems (ARS) facilitate audience engagement in a lecture by providing each attendee a small keypad with which they respond to questions posed by the lecturer. Responses are relayed via infrared or radio frequencies to a computer that integrates responses and displays them immediately in a PowerPoint™ presentation. Audience members can also be asked to use their cell phones to text in their responses, or to ask new questions of their own. Mobile devices can accomplish the same purpose with instant messaging or social media tools like Twitter. An entirely different approach to lecture interactivity might ask each attendee to link to a common website with their laptop or tablet computer and then work collaboratively and interactively on a variety of projects.

When to Use

Computer-supported audience engagement will be most useful when teaching a large audience; for smaller audiences verbal interactions might be more appropriate. An effective, interactive non-PowerPoint™ lecture probably need *not* be altered just to use a PowerPoint™- enabled ARS. Audiences may become complacent with ARS if they are overused.

Table 10.6 Tips for using audience response systems	Keep questions short and simple, and use ≤5 response options
	Use questions to emphasize key points and stimulate discussion
	Allow time for (and encourage) discussion of answers
	Rehearse, preferably in proposed location
	Provide clear instructions to audience
	Do not overuse

How to Use

Audience response questions should be short, simple, clearly written, and typically employ five or fewer response options. Questions should be used sparingly in the presentation – predominately to emphasize key points. Since the whole purpose is to encourage audience interaction, questions should be designed to stimulate discussion and time should be budgeted to permit such discussion (i.e., of the answers received). Transitions (introducing the question, presenting responses, initiating discussion, and then resuming the lecture) should be rehearsed. When lecturing in a new venue the system (commercial ARS, cell phone, mobile device, etc.) should be tested well in advance to ensure that everything works properly. If the audience is unfamiliar with the approach you will need to provide clear instructions (e.g., on how to use the keypad or text in their questions) and perhaps provide a practice question at the start. When teaching the same learners over time (e.g., a medical school course) consider tracking individual responses (e.g., through an assigned keypad, tracked phone number, or Twitter account). Table 10.6 summarizes these recommendations.

As with all technologies, ARS can be overused. Do not let fascination with the capabilities of technology take precedence over effective instructional design.

Video

What It Is

Video recordings for instructional purposes can range from brief clips integrated into lectures to full length feature films. Videoconferencing can allow a teacher at one location to reach an audience at another. Video archives or podcasts of lectures are increasingly commonplace. This section will deal primarily with the first of these uses, namely the use of video as an instructional technique.

When to Use

Video can be judiciously used to enhance any teaching activity. It can "reveal" the remote (separated by barriers of distance), the invisible (such as microscopic events or abstract concepts), and the inaccessible (unavailable due to risk or infeasibility). However, when experiences (such as lab experiments, patients, and procedures) are visible and accessible it makes sense to encounter them in person. Copyright issues should be considered before using video produced by others.

How to Use

In using video, it is critical to first define the purpose. Video can be used to provide an overview or stimulate interest at the beginning of a course; to demonstrate principles, concepts, skills, procedures, or positive or negative role models; or as a "trigger" to self-assessment and critical reflection. Your purpose will define the type of clip, the length, and most importantly the way in which you use the material. A teacher may occasionally wish to show a full-length film, but more often short clips – preferably less than 5 min in length – will be more appropriate.

If learners are not encouraged to think before, during, and after the video the exercise will become a passive process (=ineffective learning). Careful planning will prevent this problem. Before starting the video, it often helps to describe the context: the plot (especially if showing an excerpt from a longer film), the characters, and the setting. It is usually appropriate to provide an overview of what viewers will see and what they might learn, although in some instances this information might be deliberately withheld. It is always important to provide a specific objective and/or task to focus learners' attention. For example, before watching a video of a patient-physician you might suggest learners watch for specific events; attend to dialogue, body language, or emotions; identify underlying assumptions, principles, or paradigms; or reflect on their own reactions and perspectives. Likewise, before watching a video demonstrating a procedure you could ask learners to pay particular attention to a specific step, notice the sequence of steps, or look for errors. Consider pausing the video midway to recap what has happened or ask learners to predict ensuing events, or try turning down the sound and narrating events. Discussion following the video is often helpful.

Digital cameras have changed the landscape for developing new video clips. Anyone with a smartphone can now capture an event and share this via email or YouTube. Freely-available software makes the editing of clips quick and easy. Instructors can use this to develop their own clips rather than relying on pre-existing video. Learners could also video record themselves in, for example, role playing with another student, interacting with a standardized patient, performing a procedure, or giving an oral presentation. This video might then be reviewed one-on-one or (cautiously, and with permission) as a group as a stimulus for self-assessment, reflection, and formative feedback. Such assignments could be included as part of a distance-learning online course. Table 10.7 summarizes these recommendations.

Other Educational Technologies and Conclusions

This chapter could not begin to address all of the technologies available to educators today. Technologies such as overhead projectors, 35 mm slides, whiteboards and black boards, and printed materials are probably familiar to educators. Newer

Table 10.7 Tips for using video

Have a clear purpose – why are you using this clip?
Reveal remote, invisible, or inaccessible
Activate prior knowledge
Demonstrate principle/concept/skill/procedure
Trigger for discussion, self-assessment, reflection, attitude change
Set the context (plot, characters, situation); consider providing an overview
Focus attention: define objective (what can be learned) and/or task in advance
Keep clips focused (typically <5 min)
Encourage learners to think
Pause to recap, discuss, predict next events
Don't infringe copyright

technologies include virtual microscopy, virtual cadaver dissection, and simulations of various kinds. Teachers are also using clinical technologies to enhance their teaching; for example, some medical schools perform whole body CT scans of cadavers prior to anatomy lab dissection.

Given these technologies and others not mentioned (and not yet invented!), educators are faced with an ever-growing toolbox from which to select specific instructional approaches. It is easy to become enamored with one or more technologies and forget the big picture. Educational technologies are only tools to help learners learn more effectively. Those who wield these tools should not only be skilled in their use, but must know when to use each one and when a different tool is needed.

References

Bordage G (1994) Elaborated knowledge: a key to successful diagnostic thinking. Acad Med 69:883–885

Clark RC, Mayer RE (2007) E-learning and the science of instruction, 2nd edn. Pfeiffer, San Francisco

Dewey J (1913) Interest and effort in education. Houghton Mifflin, Boston

Jonassen DH (2000) Computers as mindtools for schools: engaging critical thinking, 2nd edn. Merrill Prentice Hall, Upper Saddle River

Jones C, Shao B (2011) The net generation and digital natives: implications for higher education. Higher Education Academy, York

Merrill MD (2002) First principles of instruction. Educ Technol Res Dev 50(3):43–59

Summary Report of the 2006 AAMC Colloquium on Educational Technology (2007) Effective use of educational technology in medical education. Association of American Medical Colleges, Washington, DC. https://services.aamc.org/publications

For Further Reading General Principles

Clark RC, Mayer RE (2007) E-learning and the science of instruction, 2nd edn. Pfeiffer, San Francisco

Merrill MD (2002) First principles of instruction. Educ Technol Res Dev 50(3):43–59

Summary Report of the 2006 AAMC Colloquium on Educational Technology (2007) Effective use of educational technology in medical education. Association of American Medical Colleges, Washington, DC. https://services.aamc.org/publications

Curriculum Repositories

Health Education Assets Library (HEAL) HYPERLINK http://www.healcentral.org, www.healcentral.org

Med EdPORTAL http://www.aamc.org/mededportal, www.aamc.org/mededportal

Merlot http://www.merlot.org, www.merlot.org

Computer-Assisted Learning

Cook DA, Dupras DM (2004) A practical guide to developing effective web-based learning. J Gen Intern Med 19:698–707

Ellaway R, Masters K (2008) AMEE Guide 32: e-Learning in medical education Part 1: Learning, teaching and assessment. Med Teach 30:455–473; Part 2: Technology, management and design. Med Teach 30:474–489

Ruiz JG, Cook DA, Levinson AJ (2009) Computer animations in medical education: a critical literature review. Med Educ 43:838–846

Online Communities

Gray K, Annabell L, Kennedy G (2010) Medical students' use of Facebook to support learning: insights from four case studies. Med Teach 32:971–976

Sandars J (2006a) Twelve tips for effective online discussions in continuing medical education. Med Teach 28:591–593

Sandars J (2006b) Twelve tips for using blogs and wikis in medical education. Med Teach 28:680–682

Just-In-Time Learning

Cook DA, Sorensen KJ, Wilkinson JM, Berger RA (2013) Barriers and decisions when answering clinical questions at the point of care: a grounded theory study. JAMA Intern Med 173:1962–1969

Virtual Patients

Cook DA, Triola MM (2009) Virtual patients: a critical literature review and proposed next steps. Med Educ 43:303–311

Huwendiek S, Reichert F, Bosse HM et al (2009) Design principles for virtual patients: a focus group study among students. Med Educ 43:580–588

Portfolios

Driessen E, van Tartwijk J, van der Vleuten C, Wass V (2007) Portfolios in medical education: why do they meet with mixed success? A systematic review. Med Educ 41:1224–1233

Educational Games

Tobias S, Fletcher JD (eds) (2011) Computer games and instruction. Information Age Publishing, Charlotte

Young MF, Slota S et al (2012) Our princess is in another castle: a review of trends in serious gaming for education. Rev Educ Res 82(1):61–89

Presentation Software

Holzl J (1997) Twelve tips for effective powerpoint presentations for the technologically challenged. Med Teach 19:175–179

Audience Response Systems

Robertson LJ (2000) Twelve tips for using computerised interactive audience response system. Med Teach 22:237–239

Video

Mitchell K Videography for educators. Available via http://edcommunity.apple.com/ali/story. php?itemID=365. Cited 9 Oct 2007

Chapter 11
Teaching to Develop Scientific Engagement in Medical Students

Peter G.M. de Jong and Aviad Haramati

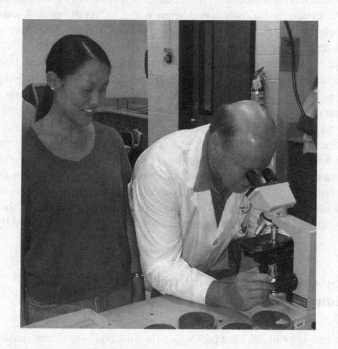

Abstract Scientific engagement refers to an attitude of the individual towards science and a specific way of thinking. This chapter emphasizes the importance of scientific engagement in medical students and provides some suggestions for how you, the

P.G.M. de Jong, Ph.D. (✉)
Leiden University Medical Center, Leiden, The Netherlands
e-mail: p.g.m.de_jong@lumc.nl

A. Haramati, Ph.D.
Georgetown University Medical Center, Washington, DC, USA

K.N. Huggett and W.B. Jeffries (eds.), *An Introduction to Medical Teaching*,
DOI 10.1007/978-94-017-9066-6_11, © Springer Science+Business Media Dordrecht 2014

teacher, can stimulate that engagement. It is important that we train scientifically minded students who are capable of performing research in a clinical research environment as well as capable of understanding, appraising and applying the research of others into their future health care position.

What Is Scientific Engagement?

Scientific engagement refers to an attitude of the individual towards science and a specific way of thinking. Scientific engagement should not be confused with scientific skills. A skill is a technical ability that can be taught, practiced, and assessed to determine if the student has mastered it. Examples are performing a statistical analysis, or conducting a laboratory procedure. Scientific engagement is something different. At its core is curiosity about science and habits of mind. A student with excellent technical scientific skills but no engagement will never become a successful research scientist or a passionate science educator.

Scientific engagement or attitude is something that can be modeled, internalized, practiced, and developed to a certain extent, depending on the personal characteristics of the individual. The reality is that many incoming medical students have had limited or no experience with scientific work, only a vague concept of the world of research, and significant misperceptions of what constitutes scientific research. Yet, medicine has its foundation in the scientific method and new information is discovered and reported at an astounding rate. Treatments evolve and become refined as more information becomes available. Since the quality of health care is dependent on scientific advances, it is worth the effort to expose students to this completely different way of thinking and working, and offer them the exciting opportunity to not only get acquainted with science, but to get enthused by it.

Why Is Scientific Engagement Important for a Medical Student?

Physicians and other health care professionals must confront the increasingly rapid production of new knowledge in the sciences fundamental to medicine (AAMC-HHMI report 2009). It is difficult to stay abreast of these new advancements in post-graduate education programs; doctors themselves struggle to keep up-to-date in their own field of expertise. Physicians are expected to find, appraise and understand new information from scientific publications. As Vandiver and Walsh describe, medical students need to understand and must learn to conduct scientific research in order to appraise experimental results when they become physicians (Vandiver and Walsch 2010). Another view has been expressed by Ludmerer, who posited that a medical diagnosis and a researcher's hypothesis are very much similar: both must be critically tested on their value (Ludmerer 2010). This is the primary reason to help our students develop a scientific way of thinking.

Therefore, we need to offer our students not only scientific knowledge and technical skills, but also to teach them the habit of mind to ask questions and integrate new scientific discoveries into their future medical practice. Engaging students for conducting research results in academically minded students who are ready to pursue research in the future, and also leads to future clinicians who are capable of understanding, appraising and applying the research of others, even if they are not looking for an academic research career (Jacobs and Cross 1995; Lawson McLean et al. 2013; Dekker 2011).

What Is It Exactly That We Want to Teach?

When we talk about fostering critical attitude, scientific curiosity and habit of mind, we are sure that many medical educators understand what we mean. However, it turns out to be very difficult to define exactly what it is. What must students learn in order to achieve the scientific engagement we are advocating? In practice, it turns out to be very difficult to describe. As an example, consider the Tuning Project of the MEDINE Thematic Network for Medical Education in Europe (http://www.tuning-medicine.com/). In this project, members of the task forces reached consensus regarding learning outcomes and competencies for undergraduate medical degree programs in Europe. These outcomes are expressed in 12 major "Level 1" outcomes, each being further defined by "Level 2" outcomes. The two science-related Level 1 outcomes are *"Apply the principles, skills and knowledge of evidence-based medicine"* and *"Ability to apply scientific principles, method and knowledge to medical practice and research."* The first outcome has some Level 2 sub-domains, like conducting a literature search and critical appraisal of the literature, but the second outcome has no Level 2 outcomes at all. Apparently, the task force members could not agree on that level of detail for those sub-domains, perhaps because faculty from individual countries or schools wished to define their own level of competencies in scientific research education.

Although there seems to be no real consensus on scientific engagement, we can delineate three aspects that should be kept in mind when teaching in this area.

Stimulation of Curiosity and an Inquiring Mind

In a research context, curiosity is the basis of scientific research and endeavor. In several studies this quality scored high among attributes that graduates should possess, as judged not only by experts but also by students and patients (Laidlaw et al. 2012; Rabinowitz et al. 2004). Once students discover, through experience, that actively searching for new knowledge in science can lead to enormous progress in health care, they will become more curious.

Ability to Critically Appraise Data

This skill is generally recognized as essential for medical students and physicians (Laidlaw et al. 2012). It is extremely important that a physician is able to analyze and critically evaluate data that are presented by others in the literature, or found in experimental setup, or returned in the form of laboratory results. This is especially relevant when students discover that the data presented sometimes differ from presented conclusions, and it will stimulate them to become more critical.

Participation and Involvement of Students

As soon as students get involved, whether in pursuing answers to questions that they raise in class, or by participating in an actual research project, they will become more engaged in science. Engaging students is not something to talk about in curricular committees, but rather something that should occur every day in the classroom or lecture hall. It is something that must be experienced.

The First Step in Student Engagement: Fostering Scientific Curiosity

Many of our students have come to expect that the learning setting in medical school, especially in the biomedical science courses, is where faculty transmit information to the students. There is an expectation many students have of receiving complete, annotated handouts, distributed sets of PowerPoint© presentation slides, audio and video capture of the sessions, all in the hope that the pertinent "facts" have appeared somewhere for the student to internalize and prepare to regurgitate on the examination. Quite a few of our faculty actually believe that is their role, as well. And yet, does the amassing of facts constitute "education"? What about understanding and application?

Lambert and colleagues very clearly articulated the goals of science education in medical school: "… *to provide students with a broad, solid foundation applicable to medicine, a deep understanding of the scientific method, and the attitudes and skills needed to apply new knowledge to patient care throughout their careers"* (Lambert et al. 2010). How do the students get a "solid foundation" and what constitutes "deep understanding"? To answer these questions, it is helpful to consider what Regehr and Norman wrote, *"True understanding […] is defined not simply by the quantity of information a person possesses, but by the extent to which this information is organized into a coherent, mutually supportive network of concepts and examples"* (Regehr and Norman 1996). In other words, the ability to use scientific information and apply scientific reasoning and principles reflects true understanding of science.

To that end, the teaching of science has moved in many institutions to incorporate case-based teaching in the form of problem-based learning or team-based learning. However, the essence here is not the method itself, but the approach. In each instance, students are asked to work with their peers and develop questions and learning issues after reviewing a particular case or considering a set of laboratory values. In other words, they are faced with getting beyond facts to the key questions and gaps in their knowledge. This we believe fosters scientific curiosity: the recognition that there is a puzzle to be solved, information to be searched, and not simply delivered to them. The student has the opportunity to solve the problem by seeking the answer, as opposed to having the facts before the question has appeared.

The importance of scientific curiosity was underscored by Dyche and Epstein: *"Medical educators should balance the teaching of facts, techniques and protocols with approaches that help students cultivate and sustain curiosity and wonder in the context-rich often ambiguous world of clinical medicine"* (Dyche and Epstein 2011).

A second aspect, that Dyche and Epstein allude to, is the notion that biomedical science is not always clear and exact; it can be ambiguous and uncertain. There are limitations to our current knowledge, which sets the stage for student engagement in pursuing new knowledge. But the first step is to be curious, something that requires some planning and patience on the part of the teacher.

In addition, to be successful, the environment must be conducive to learning and exploring. Typically in a large lecture hall, students are reluctant to answer a question in front of hundreds of students for fear of being wrong or unqualified. However, the instructor can create a safe, inviting and respectful environment by emphasizing that the answers students provide are in fact "hypothesis testing." That is, possibilities that should be explored further. And instead of acknowledging an answer as "correct" or "incorrect", the teacher could follow on the student's response by asking "what made you think that"? This way the discussion centers on the thought process more than being right or wrong.

The Second Step in Student Engagement: How to Involve Students in Scientific Research Projects?

Once their curiosity has been stimulated, students will be motivated to seek answers, sometimes by engaging in new scientific research projects. This leads to the second step of student engagement: the independent research project. To be successful, students need to learn fundamental research competencies and we need to train them in the process of scientific critical, inquisitive and analytical thinking. The way this scientific training is incorporated in the curriculum differs from country to country and from institution to institution (Jenkins et al. 2003). In some medical schools scientific research is a mandatory part of the core undergraduate curriculum, while in other schools training in this field is offered as an elective or not offered at all. In 2012 the online journal *Medical Science Educator* published a special issue on student research projects in scientific research for undergraduate medical students (Medical Science Educator 2013). The content of the issue reflects the diversity in how this topic is handled by institutions from all over the world. A large European study organized by MEDINE (Thematic Network on Medical Education in Europe) in 2006–2007 showed that among 91 surveyed medical schools, 75 % of the schools did offer research courses to medical students, but less than 10 % of the students select this option (Van Schravendijk et al. 2013). This low number suggests that engagement does not simply occur, but has to be stimulated in some way. Therefore, it is very important that medical schools offer integrated research programs. Students need opportunities to practice their research skills by performing real research projects and to be challenged by scientifically exploring medicine.

In the traditional view, the process of learning research skills can be divided into four stages as described by Healey (2005). The first phase is a research-led phase, where students learn about current research, typically in large group class settings. The second phase is a more research-oriented stage, where students are introduced to research skills and inquiry and survey techniques. They learn procedural skills, declarative knowledge and comprehension in research design and methods, interpretation of simple to moderately complex literature, fundamental principles of epidemiology and evidence based practice. These two phases generally apply passive teaching methods, often in large groups and in many cases non-authentic (i.e., not related to medicine) settings. The third phase is more research-based where students undertake simple research projects themselves. They can practice the skills by performing mentored student research projects. And in phase 4 the student conducts an independent research project under supervision of a tutor, eventually becoming a physician-scientist or health practitioner-scientist. Phase 3 and 4 are much more participatory and active ways of learning by doing.

It is known that active and authentic learning approaches are more effective in mastering skills than passive ways (Vandiver and Walsh 2010). To optimize this, we feel the traditional sequence as described above should be modified. Vereijken et al. describe a case in which students already in the beginning of medical school are actively engaged in a research project that is conducted with the complete cohort of more than 300 students working together on one research question (Vereijken et al. 2013). In this scenario, the students immediately proceeded from phase 1 to phase 3–4 in the Healey model. Another example, described by Gruis and Langenhoff, involved students in research starting on day one of their biomedical research curriculum (Gruis and Langenhoff 2013). We believe that these innovative ways of teaching are valuable and ought to be adopted in an effort to foster scientific engagement in our students.

Creating opportunities for students to pursue scientific research in the undergraduate medical curriculum promotes enthusiasm for scientific research and scientific engagement of the students. A possible parameter to measure this effect is the number of publications after graduation. Several studies show that students do publish their work, and that those who experienced active and authentic scientific research in an early stage of the curriculum tend to have a higher publication rate after graduation (Dyrbye et al. 2008; van Eyk et al. 2010; Reinders et al. 2005).

Tips for Involving Students into Scientific Research

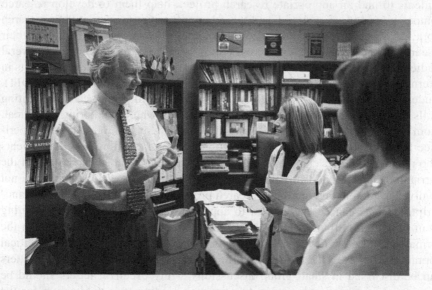

Lawson McLean et al. published 12 tips for teachers to encourage student engagement in academic medicine (Lawson McLean et al. 2013). These 12 recommendations are based on a review of the literature and on their own personal experiences. We are reflecting on those suggestions here and encourage you to adapt one or more in your own teaching.

Not every medical school offers opportunities for students to experience research. In that case consider having faculty offer projects, small or large, mandatory or voluntary, to give students some experience in this field. Even small projects are a good start. Try to integrate the teaching of practical research techniques and laboratory skills with actual opportunities to do some research, to make sure the students see the purpose of these techniques. In the case research projects are available, include students in the full process of a research project, including proposal writing, fundraising and discussing ethical issues before the project starts. Often students are asked to contribute to a small component of an ongoing project; this makes them miss the opportunity to experience the entirety of the project. That overall perspective is vitally important in order to develop an engagement in research. Undergraduate research electives can be offered to give interested students a chance to experience research in an early stage of the curriculum. Experiences show that the number of students considering a research career increases by offering these learning opportunities (Bahner et al. 2012; Houlden et al. 2004). Consider involving students in international research collaborations or exchange programs. These offer students an exciting experience to learn and work in an academic setting but in a different environment and a different culture.

Teachers can support students on an individual basis. Mentorship can provide students an inspirational role model for a medical researcher. Mentors can help students to find an appropriate research project, help them to develop research competencies not yet achieved, and to find opportunities to present their research work. As a teacher you should encourage students to present the results of their research project as a conference presentation or in a journal publication. Several studies demonstrate that students value the opportunity to publish their results in international journals (Griffin and Hindocha 2011; de Oliveira et al. 2011). Students feel it is important to publish, but often lack adequate academic writing skills to successfully author a manuscript. This is where mentoring is critical. From the literature we know that students who had substantial research experience before graduation publish more articles after graduation than the students who did not (Reinders et al. 2005). Apparently publishing at an early stage of the curriculum engages students for scientific work. But even when students are not involved in conducting their own research project and collecting data for a manuscript, students can be encouraged to appraise research in the field by inviting them to write a critique of or a letter that comments on published work, in the format of a "Letter to the Editor". In this way students develop their critical appraisal skills as well as their scientific writing skills. To start with, the letters can be discussed in small group discussions. Truly excellent letters should be considered for actual submission to a journal, leading to a publication for the student. Encourage students to attend research meetings, journal clubs, symposia and conferences, to get them motivated by hearing others presenting their work. If costs are a potential barrier, consider setting up a fund where students can apply for a small grant to offset costs.

As academic research and teaching are closely connected, students also develop an academic mindset from teaching others. As their teaching mentor, you can develop opportunities for students to teach, and help them to improve their teaching skills through courses and workshops. Several medical schools offer elective courses in medical teaching to prepare the students for that future role. We strongly believe that being involved in scientific research and academic teaching can reinforce each other resulting in better critical thinking and higher motivation. It also raises students' awareness about possible future academic career opportunities in research and education. Having researchers from outside your institution participating in your course, either in person or through a video link, also helps students broaden their understanding of research and the potential benefits of an academic career.

Fostering Scientific Engagement in Students: Case Studies

Following below are examples from our own institutions of approaches that offer a scientific experience to medical or biomedical sciences students aimed at increasing their scientific engagement.

Example 1: Writing and Critiquing a Scientific Mini-Review: A Lesson in Peer-Review (Georgetown University)

One of the more innovative activities that fosters scientific thinking and curiosity occurs in the first year module at Georgetown that covers: *Sexual Development and Reproduction (SDR)* directed by Dr. G. Ian Gallicano. One of the requirements for this module is that students (in groups of 4) must write a scientific mini-review on a topic they select from a list of possibilities. On the first day of class, the purpose of writing this paper is described to the class and the format and assignments are made. Thus, the team must work together on this activity using a clear rubric and completing the task in 12 days. The papers are submitted electronically by group number to the module director, who then assigns them to other groups to conduct a peer-review (much like any review of a journal article). The anonymity is maintained, as only the module director knows which students are in which groups. The critiquing group has 5 days to complete the peer-review (following a defined rubric and evaluation form) and the original writing group can rebut the elements of the critique to the module director. Sixty percent of the points are awarded for writing the paper and 40 % for the critique (including an assessment of individual author contributions). The highest scoring papers (about seven) are bound and held in the medical school's library and several are submitted for publication. In the 4 years that this activity has been part of the module, over 10 papers have been published in a peer-reviewed journal. This task has been challenging for the students, but also very rewarding and most report that it increased their interest and enthusiasm for the subject matter.

Example 2: Critically Appraising Drug Advertisements (Leiden University Medical School)

Leiden Medical School has a modern curriculum defined by competency-based educational outcomes. Besides teaching the sciences fundamental to medicine, special attention is paid to the personal development of competencies in longitudinal programs along the entire 6-year curriculum, integrated in the regular courses. One of these programs focusses on the academic and scientific development of students by engaging students in scientific research and academic scholarship.

As part of this program a 3-week collaborative research course is offered in the second year with a full class size of approximately 300 students. The goal of the course is to foster a scientific mindset and to encourage participation in science by offering some theory regarding research study design, critical reading, statistics, data analysis and presentation of outcomes, all related to one central research question posed: *"What percentage of the clinical trials referred to in drug advertisements accurately support the claims made in the advertisement?"*. To answer this question, all students together rate 150 preselected randomized controlled trials (RCT) and the pharmaceutical advertisements in which they were referenced. Every student works on only two of these RCTs, and every RCT is reviewed by four different students.

The students enter the data in an online database on which statistical analyses are performed. As a result of this course format, the entire class rates 150 RCTs as if they were one virtual researcher. The results of the analysis are discussed in class. In this case, the conclusion of the study is that a solid RCT reference does not automatically support the claim made in the advertisement. From this exercise the students learn that critical appraisal of the literature is a necessary skill for medical doctors, with clear implications for treatment. And by collaborating as an entire class working on a single research question, engagement for scientific research increases.

The group in Leiden did several experiments with a full class size group to increase engagement in and awareness of scientific research, of which results have been published (Dekker and de Craen 2009; Vereijken et al 2013). Their experiences might offer you inspiration for what you might do in your own course.

Example 3: Introducing Research Practice on Day 1 of the Program (Leiden University School for Biomedical Sciences)

Students at Leiden School of Biomedical Sciences in the Netherlands go through the full process of conducting a literature search, extracting the information needed and presenting the results in an introductory course in the very first week of the curriculum. The goal of the course is to immediately engage students in science and to let them experience what research is all about. From past experiences it was known that giving training in scientific skills alone is not successful. When students cannot see the relevance of the training they receive, it is very difficult to motivate them. Secondly, the acquired research skills were often forgotten by the time these were needed in research projects later in the curriculum. Therefore the course has been redesigned into its current format. The key change has been to integrate the scientific training with biomedical lectures and small group activities in a specific field of science. For this specific course the topic of "skin cancer" has been chosen. This topic has relevance in the daily life of the students or their families, which was felt to be a motivating factor.

The course consists of five main elements, and all activities in the course are concentrated around a realistic research question in the field of skin cancer that students have to work on and solve (Fig. 11.1). In the first step, skin cancer is discussed in detail. It represents the basic biomedical elements that a researcher will encounter. The second step is an orientation on the research questions. Through an interactive mind map session, the students are encouraged to broaden their minds on the scope of the research questions, the research goals and how to achieve them. This process is reinforced in a teleconferenced meeting with a researcher from another research institute somewhere in the world. In this session, the students get the opportunity to ask questions and discuss topics with that researcher. With a clear view on the biomedical content (skin cancer) and the questions they have to solve (mind map session), the students enter step 3. In this phase, students learn to formulate an effective literature search strategy and to perform a database search in

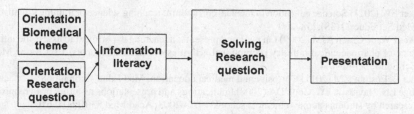

Fig. 11.1 Layout of the course (From Gruis and Langenhoff 2013, with permission)

PubMed. From this point on, students work in pairs to solve one of the seven research questions available, using the information and the skills they learned in the days before. They meet in small groups to discuss their progress and questions under guidance of an experienced tutor/researcher. Finally, the students present their results in pairs to the other students in the group. This presentation must be organized in a scientific way to let them experience how a researcher is expected to present data. Grading of the course is based on the scientific quality of the presentation and the quality of the literature search that was performed.

The experiences with this problem-oriented, integrated course on scientific and academic skills are very positive. Students get engaged in the field of skin cancer and more importantly for research in general. The presentations clearly show the students acquired a good understanding of scientific research. This first course is a strong base for the following courses in the curriculum and triggers the students' curiosity regarding biomedical research.

Conclusions

In this chapter we have tried to emphasize the importance of scientific engagement in medical students and provided some suggestions for how you, the teacher, can stimulate that engagement. It is important that we train scientifically minded students who are capable of performing research in a clinical research environment as well as capable of understanding, appraising and applying the research of others into their future health care position. We hope that this discussion and examples are helpful for you as a teacher in the exciting environment of medical science education.

References

Bahner I, Somboonwit C, Pross S, Collins RJ, Saporta S (2012) Teaching science through biomedical research in an elective curriculum. Med Sci Educ 22(3S):143–146

de Oliveira NA, Luz MR, Saraiva RM, Alves LA (2011) Student views of research training programmes in medical schools. Med Educ 45(7):748–755

Dekker FW (2011) Science education in medical curriculum: teaching science or training scientists? Med Sci Educ 21(3S):258–260

Dekker FW, de Craen AJM (2009) On pens and presents: a teaching experiment to assess the influence of pharmaceutical industry promotional activities on medical students. J Int Assoc Med Sci Educ 19:142–144

Dyche L, Epstein RM (2011) Curiosity and medical education. Med Educ 45:663–668

Dyrbye LN, Davidson LW, Cook DA (2008) Publications and presentations resulting from required research by students at mayo medical school, 1976–2003. Acad Med 83(6):604–610

Griffin MF, Hindocha S (2011) Publication practices of medical students at British medical schools: experience, attitudes and barriers to publish. Med Teach 33(1):e1–e8

Gruis NA, Langenhoff JM (2013) Increasing first year Student's attitude and understanding towards biomedical research. Med Sci Educ 23(1S):148–153

Healey M (2005) Linking research and teaching: exploring disciplinary spaces and the role of inquiry-based learning. In: Barnett R (ed) Reshaping the university: new relationships between research, scholarship and teaching. McGraw Hill/Open University Press, Maidenhead/New York, pp 67–78

Houlden RL, Raja JB, Collier CP, Clark AF, Waugh JM (2004) Medical students' perceptions of an undergraduate research elective. Med Teach 26:659–661

Jacobs CD, Cross PC (1995) The value of medical student research: the experience at Stanford University School of medicine. Med Educ 29(5):342–346

Jenkins A, Breen R, Lindsay R (2003) Reshaping teaching in higher education: linking teaching with research. Kogan Page Limited, London

Laidlaw A, Aiton J, Struthers J, Guild S (2012) Developing research skills in medical students: AMEE guide No. 69. Med Teach 34:754–771

Lambert DR, Lurie SJ, Lyness JM, Ward DS (2010) Standardizing and personalizing science in medical education. Acad Med 85:356–362

Lawson Mclean A, Saunders C, Palani Velu P, Iredale J, Hor K, Russel CD (2013) Twelve tips for teachers to encourage student engagement in academic medicine. Med Teach 35:549–554

Ludmerer K (2010) Understanding the Flexner report. Acad Med 85(2):193–196

Rabinowitz D, Reis S, van Raalte R, Alroy G, Ber R (2004) Development of a physician attributes database as a resource for medical education, professionalism and student evaluation. Med Teach 26(2):160–165

Regehr G, Norman GR (1996) Issues in cognitive psychology: implications for professional education. Acad Med 71:988–1001

Reinders JJ, Kropmans TJ, Cohen-Schotanus J (2005) Extracurricular research experience of medical students and their scientific output after graduation. Med Educ 39:237

Scientific Foundations for Future Physicians (2009) AAMC-HHMI report, Washington DC, USA

Supplement on Student Research Projects (2013) Med Sci Educ 23(1S)

Van Eyk HJ, Hooiveld MHW, van Leeuwen TN, van der Wurff BLJ, de Craen AJM, Dekker FW (2010) Scientific output of Dutch medical students. Med Teach 32:231–235

Van Schravendijk C, März R, Garcia-Seoane J (2013) Exploring the integration of the biomedical research component in undergraduate medical education. Med Teach 35:e1243–e1251

Vandiver DM, Walsh JA (2010) Assessing autonomous learning in research methods courses: implementing the student-driven research project. Act Learn High Educ 11:31–42

Vereijken MWC, Kruidering-Hall M, de Jong PGM, de Beaufort AJ, Dekker FW (2013) Scientific education early in the curriculum using a constructivist approach on learning. PME. doi:10.1007/s40037-013-0072-1

Further Reading

Cruser A, Dubin B, Brown SK, Bakken LL, Licciardone JC, Podawiltz AL, Bulik RJ (2009) Biomedical research competencies for osteopathic medical students. Osteopath Med Prim Care 3:10

Dekker FW, Halbesma N, Zeestraten EA, Vogelpoel EM, Blees MT, de Jong PGM (2009) Scientific training in the Leiden medical school preclinical curriculum to prepare students for their research projects. J Int Assoc Med Sci Educ 19(2S):2–6

des Cruser A, Brown SK, Ingram JR, Papa F, Podawiltz AL, Lee D, Knox V (2012) Practitioner research literacy skills in undergraduate medical education: thinking globally, acting locally. Med Sci Educ 22(3):162–184

MacDougall M, Riley SC (2010) Initiating undergraduate medical students into communities of research practise: what do supervisors recommend? BMC Med Educ 10:83

Patrício M, Harden RM (2010) The bologna process – a global vision for the future of medical education. Med Teach 32:305–315

Simons M, Elen J (2007) The research teaching nexus and education through research: an exploration of ambivalences. Stud High 32:617–631

Solomon SS, Tom SC, Pichert J, Wasserman D, Powers AC (2003) Impact of medical student research in the development of physician-scientists. J Invest Med 51(3):149–156

Supplement on Core-Competencies in Scientific Research for Undergraduate Medical Education (2012) Med Sci Educ 22(3S)

Chapter 12
Designing a Course

Susan J. Pasquale and N. Kevin Krane

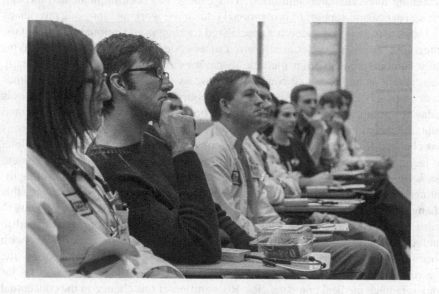

Abstract This chapter discusses the principles of overall course design, emphasizing the concept of backward design: outlining what should students be able to do by the end of the course, and then determining what they must learn in order to achieve the target levels of knowledge and performance. From this specification will come the course goals and objectives, which must be consistent with the overall curricular goals and objectives. Learning resources must be identified, and the appropriate

S.J. Pasquale, Ph.D. (✉)
Johnson & Wales University, Providence, RI, USA
e-mail: susan.pasquale@jwu.edu

N.K. Krane, MD, FACP
Tulane University School of Medicine, New Orleans, LA, USA

K.N. Huggett and W.B. Jeffries (eds.), *An Introduction to Medical Teaching*,
DOI 10.1007/978-94-017-9066-6_12, © Springer Science+Business Media Dordrecht 2014

teaching methods for the course must be determined. Finally, but no less important, appropriate assessment and feedback approaches must be selected.

Introduction

Medical school has traditionally consisted of a set of independent courses that future physicians were expected to pass to receive their medical degree and advance into postgraduate medical education. Currently, however, medical education is evolving in a way that assures that students will be well-prepared for their next level of learning by requiring them to demonstrate that they have developed the necessary knowledge, skills and attitudes for residency. As a result, the medical curriculum is becoming integrated and centralized. This change has been implemented through the assistance and support of professional educators, working alongside physicians and scientists, who have acquired specialized training in educational fundamentals. Integrated "courses," sometimes referred to as systems "blocks or modules," typically combine content from multiple disciplines each of which had traditionally been taught as an individual course. The process of integration across disciplines has completely changed the definition of a "course" as it exists in medical schools today. In many schools today, one would be challenged to still find traditional courses labeled as biochemistry, physiology, or pathology. The instructional focus has changed from "teaching," in terms of conveying the basic facts of a discipline, to facilitating student learning. This transition has led to the integration of content across disciplines, as well as across basic and clinical sciences, as a means of facilitating and streamlining the learning process for adult learners. Furthermore, this change has resulted in growing awareness that there is much more for students to learn than "just" facts. As a result, the aim of medical education has widened to include the development of attitudinal and behavioral competencies along with specific knowledge, often using the competencies initially developed by the Accreditation Council on Graduate Medical Education (ACGME) as the basis for undergraduate medical competencies. Recognition of this change in the conceptual framework of medical education is essential in understanding that a given course may be presented as one of several types of learning units: a traditional discipline-based course, a set of disciplines organized into a single course, or several learning units each of which may each represent a course or may be combined into an integrated course. Regardless of the course configuration, educators must determine what students need to learn to meet the societal and institutional objectives that will assure their development of the competencies necessary for future physicians in the rapidly changing healthcare environment. Given this changing perspective on teaching and learning in medicine, if you as a junior faculty member were asked to design a course, how would you go about it? What would you do, and where would you start, to design a course for preclinical students entitled "The Kidney and Genitourinary (GU) System"?

Initial Considerations

The first step is to start at the end. Begin with *backward design*. Wiggins and McTighe (2005) emphasize that backward design is a three-stage approach. First, what do you want learners to understand and what questions will address this issue? Secondly, what methods will you use to collect evidence that students do understand and can apply what they have learned? And finally what is the learning plan and what are the learning activities that will be used? From the perspective of future physicians, think not about what you want students to know but what they should be able to do with their knowledge. How will they apply what they learn? One must start with a clear set of goals and objectives. For example, to design a Kidney/GU System Module, one might start with a goal of familiarizing students with the most important clinical problems that every physician must learn about: urinary tract infection, chronic kidney disease due to hypertension and diabetes, prostate cancer, hematuria.

Backward design begins with specifying why the course is needed by the learners. For example if the course is an educational unit on the kidney and genitourinary tract for students with limited clinical experience, you may want them to be able to know how to evaluate a patient who presents with gross hematuria. This will require that they learn the structural and physiologic basis for hematuria, diseases that present with hematuria, sufficient clinical epidemiology to understand risks of diseases in different populations, and the clinical skills necessary for history taking and examination. One should therefore be able to articulate what is the purpose of the course; why is it needed, what information will be conveyed in it that is important for the learners to acquire and what will they be able to do with this knowledge when the course is finished? To support the development of skill in applying knowledge, it is important to delineate the knowledge, skills, attitudes and behaviors that must be demonstrated at the end of the course (or other learning unit) to show that learners have achieved mastery of the content.

The primary goal of teaching is to facilitate learning; therefore, it is essential that course activities be oriented toward the process of learning. Additionally, it is important to make a distinction between theories of learning and theories of teaching. While theories of learning deal with how an individual learns, theories of teaching describe how a teacher influences learning behavior (Gage 1972, p. 73). Knowles et al. (1973, p. 17) make a further distinction by noting that learning is defined as "the process of gaining knowledge and or expertise … and … emphasizes the person in whom the change is expected to occur, [while] education emphasizes the educator." It is presumed that the learning theory subscribed to by an educator will influence his or her choice of teaching methods.

Accordingly, in order for the teacher's activities to be oriented toward the process of learning, and for the process of learning to guide our teaching practice, the teacher must address specific background information that will guide the course design.

1. Who is the learner? What knowledge, skills and attitudes will they bring to the course?

2. How many learners will there be in the course and at each session and how will you design the learning for the number of learners you have?
3. What is the venue in which you will be teaching, or in which you will choose to teach? Based on the venue, what type of learning methodologies are likely to be most effective for the content you are seeking to convey, for the level of learners that you have, and for the type of physical space you will be teaching in? There are significant differences between medical school courses that are completely classroom based and those that have laboratory or clinical experiences.

With these goals in mind, what knowledge, skills, attitudes and behaviors do you expect students to acquire? How will your module contribute to students' ability to achieve the ACGME competencies (i.e., medical knowledge, patient care, communication, practice-based learning, systems-based practice)? Knowledge of the Kidney/GU system basics can be acquired by many good texts that are available, and standardized exams can be used to assess that knowledge. On the other hand, one would want students to be able to perform a basic prostate examination (patient care), communicate the results of prostate cancer screening to a patient (communication) and be able to understand differences in the medical literature regarding the use of prostate screening tests (practice-based learning). These examples represent the first steps of backward design and indicate what to think about before beginning to design your course.

Regardless of whether the course consists of a single module (the Kidney and GU Systems), or is a more comprehensive unit of instruction combining several modules (i.e., a multisystem, mechanisms of disease course), there is a common set of educational principles necessary to maximize student learning. For the purposes of this chapter, we will refer to design of an instructional unit as design of a course. Traditionally, course design has focused on determining what knowledge or content must be learned; when students could demonstrate they knew those facts, they would advance. Because medical education is currently moving to a competency-based approach, modern course design should address not only competency in knowledge, but should also consider which other competencies, such as professionalism and communication skills, should be addressed within the course. For example, if students are learning gross anatomy by dissecting as a team, principles of communication and professionalism might easily become part of the course design. Using the second phase of backwards design, one would determine not only which competencies should be assessed, but how to do so. Using backward design provides each course with an excellent opportunity to incorporate instructional elements that will develop the skills, behaviors and attitudes necessary for the successful practice of medicine.

Establishing Goals and Objectives

Backward design requires that the instructor address what learners should be able to do with what they have learned. Identification of such performance requirements will provide the course goals. For example, at the end of a course on the Kidney and

GU System, students would know how to examine and counsel a 55 year-old man for prostate cancer screening, but one would not expect them to know chemotherapy regimens for prostate cancer. Using this approach, one can establish a comprehensive set of course objectives.

The purpose of course objectives is to let learners and others know what learners should achieve. Effective objectives are related to intended outcomes, as well as to the process for achieving those outcomes; give clear criteria for achievement; are specific and measurable, rather than broad and intangible; and focus on the learners, not the teachers (Mager 1962). Objectives should be specific, observable, measureable, attainable, realistic, learner-oriented and appropriate for the level of the learner. An objective is considered measurable when it describes something tangible. While a goal is a broad statement of the overall outcome you seek to achieve, objectives are specific statements of how you will get there and how you will know when you have achieved the objective. Generally, when each objective has been achieved the goal has been met. Thus, the objectives function as stepping stones to meeting the overall goals. It is helpful if objectives are thought of as containing five elements (Kern et al. 1998):

1. Who
2. Will do
3. How much (or how well)
4. Of what
5. By when

Another way to think of the elements is:

- Performance: Describes what the learner is expected to be able to DO
- Conditions: Describes the conditions under which the performance is expected to occur
- Criterion: Describes the level of competence that must be reached or surpassed

Goals and objectives are often related to competencies. Within medical education, competencies are skills or abilities that learners completing a program or course of study are expected to have mastered. Specific competency domains or skill sets that are fundamental to the practice of medicine, and broad in scope, have been identified by organizations such as the Institute of Medicine (IOM), Accreditation Council for Graduate Medical Education (ACGME) and Royal College of Physicians and Surgeons of Canada. Each competency is defined by a one-sentence statement, followed by an elaboration that describes the types of behavior and attitudes that reflect mastery of the competency. Goals and objectives associated with each competency help to further define that specific competency, including how the competency will be measured.

In a medical school curriculum it is usually easy to identify the learners, what they need to know and be able to apply, what information they will bring to the course and what information and skills they need to master in the course in order to proceed to the subsequent level of learning. Once this information has been determined, it is a relatively straightforward process to develop goals and objectives that will facilitate development of the requisite competencies. A competency framework serves to guide how the material in the course will be organized. If it is essential that certain knowledge be acquired and applied in a specific sequence of learning, then it also will be necessary to determine how the content will be organized and which teaching methods will be applied to ensure the content will be presented sequentially.

Identifying Learning Resources

After the initial course design has been laid out beginning with goals and objectives, one must then review the resources available for the course. Resources can include instructors, facilities, technology, teaching materials, patients, and equipment. Creative thinking can often address resource limitations. For example, many schools train fourth-year students as facilitators for small group teaching; low-fidelity simulation may be able to meet course goals instead of high-fidelity simulation; and TBL can provide active learning for a large class of students when faculty numbers are limited. In some communities, expensive facilities such as those for standardized patients or simulation may be shared.

For centuries, the primary learning resource has been the professor, who imparted essential knowledge to the students, most often in lecture form. Lecture can still be a valuable learning resource, but particularly in medical school, one of the expected outcomes is that students will develop ability in self-directed learning and application of knowledge, rather than just memorizing material to pass an examination. Learning resources, therefore, can and should include textbooks, journal articles, and material posted online by faculty to guide student learning, such as pre-recorded mini-lectures that provide an introduction or overview to material. Pre-recorded online material posted by experts outside the parent institution could be another useful resource. Additional examples of learning resources include images appropriate for the anatomical sciences or pathology, and videos that demonstrate neurologic findings or dynamic scientific processes. As technology continues to enhance educational materials, faculty must consider how to stimulate learning through newer and more dynamic learning resources.

Creating Content: Prior Knowledge and New Information

While designing the course, one should remember that a goal of learning is to assimilate new information into an existing format, or schema, located within the learner's memory. The more connections created between the new information and prior knowledge, the easier it will be for the student to remember the new information, which will become part of, and strengthened by, the connections that already exist (Svinicki 1993–1994). This is particularly true in medical education where students base their learning of pathophysiology and pathology on normal structure and function. Assuming this knowledge is learned accurately to begin with, it is important to build on this prior knowledge so that new knowledge acquired by the learner does not link to inaccurate or misconceived principles and hence an incorrect foundation of information. It is also important to recognize that, typical of adult learning behavior, the outcomes of student learning will be influenced by the prior knowledge they bring to their medical school experiences. This can be particularly challenging in the first year of medical education given that some students have advanced science degrees while other students have liberal arts degrees and have completed only the minimal requirements for medical school admission. Thus the current level of the learners' knowledge bases must be considered in helping them build on prior knowledge and skills.

Regardless of learners' incoming knowledge level, the course goals and objectives will be the same. This is a particularly important consideration in competency-based education in which students with prior experience and knowledge may be able to demonstrate competence in specific areas more quickly than their peers. One must also consider that learners have preferred ways of processing information and that many variables influence ways in which students prefer to learn. Such variables include whether students prefer to learn independently, from peers, or teachers; whether they prefer to learn through auditory, tactile, kinesthetic or visual inputs; whether they prefer information that is more detail-oriented, concrete, abstract, or combinations of these; and the characteristics of the physical environment in which they prefer to learn.

Once you have identified the knowledge, skills, and attitudes/behaviors that the learners must demonstrate to indicate mastery of the content, and once you have identified what prior learning students are bringing to your course, you can begin to determine what content will be needed to fill the gap between what learners need to know to achieve the course objectives and what they already know. As you begin to create the content, it is also helpful to seek information about the relationship between your course and the expectations of other course directors who make up the overall educational program. For example, if students in a family medicine clerkship are expected to know how to screen for prostate cancer, then the "Kidney-GU Module" must ensure that students learn the most current guidelines for using the prostate specific assay (PSA), how to discuss the PSA guidelines with patients, and how to do a prostate exam. Therefore, it will be crucial to identify what students will need to know for subsequent steps in the curriculum; and what skills they will need to master in order to proceed to the next level of knowledge and to apply that knowledge effectively.

Attention to the organization and details of a course are essential. Students expect and should be given a road map on Day 1 of the course. This road map generally takes the form of a syllabus, often provided online. Basic elements of the syllabus include: the goals and objectives of the course, the learning resources, a course schedule and how students will be evaluated. Most medical school courses tend to be very complex with faculty from many disciplines participating and using varied pedagogical styles, multiple locations, and several methods of evaluation. All of this information must be provided to students when they begin the course, typically posted on a course website which may use either commercial or institutional software. This is particularly important for clinical rotations where students must catalog their experiences, work under the supervision of residents and attendings, and receive assessment based on the observation of their clinical skills.

Teaching Methods

Thus far, the focus of this discussion has been on establishing the course content based on the overall goals of the educational program, the course objectives, and the competencies that must be achieved. Following these initial steps, one can begin to consider the pedagogy or teaching methods that will be used to promote mastery of the content, so that learners can move to the next level of learning. In determining the pedagogy, one must consider many variables, such as the course goals, the number of learners, the physical space in which the course will take place, and the resources available to deliver the course. While lecture has traditionally been considered the primary teaching/learning method, medical education has embraced the importance of self-directed and active learning as essential elements of an effective leaning process. Advances in technology have significantly changed how content can be delivered and how students prefer to learn; course directors must consider these changes. The expectation that students must attend lectures to gain knowledge is largely disappearing. Lectures still serve a valuable function in education, but technological changes and greater understanding of adult learning theory have made the lecture format and attendance at lectures less essential. In medical schools that do not utilize active learning, lectures are usually recorded and made available online in either real time or on demand. Most topics are readily available online in multiple formats via institutional and individual online posting, and the ability to create useful online videos has become surprisingly easy. Unfortunately, when assigned fewer lecture hours for their material, some faculty simply increase the amount of content in their presentations. This will overwhelm students and make the presentations even less useful. Good course design addresses the balance of lecture and non-lecture activities.

Recently, significant acceptance has been gained for techniques such as the "reverse classroom" and other in-depth learning and interactive teaching methods which require students to come prepared so that class time can be used to apply knowledge. Content delivery methods are therefore in rapid flux and the future of course content delivery appears likely to include vehicles such as Massive Open Online Courses (MOOCs). The concept of learning resources is rapidly changing. In designing courses one must take this ongoing change process into account. No longer are the course delivery resources limited to the institutional faculty; instructional resources should include those available online, both internal and external to the institution. Repositories of excellent, peer reviewed educational material are becoming more and more common at sites such as MedEdPORTAL, and course directors should be aware of these peer-reviewed materials which are often more easy to incorporate in their teaching plans than to develop new and untested material. Additional examples of peer-reviewed teaching material include those being created by specialty organizations, traditional textbooks, journal articles, and various online materials/lectures. The challenge for course directors is how best to employ principles of effective learning given the changes in medical school class size, and limited instructional resources, learner characteristics and new outcome requirements (such as competencies). Some examples of adult learning that require students to come to class prepared, work effectively with classmates, and apply knowledge to solve problems are Just-In-Time Teaching (JiTT), Problem-Based Learning (PBL), Team-Based Learning (TBL) and Simulation Learning. Each method has its own advantages and disadvantages; for example, TBL offers the advantage that one faculty member can facilitate an entire class, while PBL requires facilitators for each small group. If students need to learn clinical skills such as cardiac examination, they may benefit from working with standardized patients or a cardiac simulator.

If one thinks carefully about the goal of the learning process, or what students should be able to do when they have learned your course content, one realizes there are now many ways in which faculty can structure the content to facilitate effective learning. The fact that technology now plays a significant role in course delivery makes it necessary for course directors to be aware of both hardware and software that can improve student learning. As an example, most microscopic anatomical imaging is presented online using virtual microscopy rather than actual microscopy. Another example is simulation, which offers unique opportunities both in basic and clinical science. Although technology presents its own challenges, faculty must be prepared to incorporate some of the newer methods into their course design in order to save time, reduce contact-hour requirements, and facilitate learning for students who are accustomed to using technology.

As you begin to determine the pedagogy you will use to convey the knowledge and skills, it will be useful to review the guidelines offered by taxonomies of learning such as Bloom's (1956). Consider how the learners will need to apply the information that you provide, and in what situations they will need to apply it. For example, a scenario with standardized patients may be an ideal format for students to learn how to speak to patients about PSA screening. A low-fidelity simulator may be the simplest way for students to learn how to do the prostate exam, while a self-study, online module may provide an effective format to learn about the prostate guidelines.

Essential to this process is an awareness of the relationship between the learner's motivation and approach to learning. Intrinsic motivation has been shown to link to a deep approach to learning while extrinsic motivation links to a surface approach to learning. In designing a course, always consider how to motivate student learning. For most medical students learning fundamental basic science seems very abstract. Knowing why they are learning the content can provide needed motivation to learn in a way that will promote retention, along with the ability to recall and apply the information appropriately. In the kidney, glomerular hemodynamics may seem like an abstract and esoteric concept to students unless they are first motivated by the clinical picture of diabetic nephropathy, the most common cause of kidney failure in the United States. Learning first that the standard treatment of this disease is to alter the glomerular hemodynamics with specific drugs is an important motivating factor. Similarly, if one wanted students to learn about patient safety, one might ask a class: "Who in this class has had a family member suffer an adverse event because of a health care error?" Motivation, other than the motivation to earn a high grade on an examination is important. Mann (1999, p. 238) endorses attention to the relationship between motivation and learning, noting that the two are integrally related. "A necessary element in encouraging the shift from extrinsic to intrinsic motivation appears to be the opportunity for learners to practice a skill/task until they gain competence; satisfaction with accomplishments and competence is itself motivating, and encourages in the learner further practice and the confidence to undertake new tasks."

Medical school faculty must merge the practical aspects of what students need to be able to learn and do with the educational principles that serve as the scaffolding in creating a course. Faculty must be aware of the students' level of prior knowledge, and the abstract conceptualization of what was learned and the implications for future iterations of the same experience (i.e., what will be done differently next time). The overall goal is to facilitate the learner's progression through levels of competence representing the five stages of Miller's triangle (i.e., knows what, knows how, shows how, does, and mastery) (Dent and Harden 2009), as well as by Bloom's taxonomy of cognitive learning (Bloom 1956). Bloom's hierarchy consists of six levels of increasing difficulty or depth representing the cognitive domain are:

1. remembering (e.g., recalling or remembering the information)
2. understanding (e.g., explaining ideas or concepts)
3. applying (e.g., applying the information in a new way)
4. analyzing (e.g., calling upon relevant information; distinguishing between the different parts)
5. evaluating (e.g., comparing and evaluating plans; justifying a stand or decision).
6. creating (e.g., creating a new point of view or product)

Use of these principles is essential for constructing effective learning objectives when in the process of course design.

Assessment of Learning

Finally, assessment must be built into the initial planning of the course. An old dictum is that, if something is not worth assessing, it's not worth doing. Moreover, the assessment method must be appropriate for the learning objective and correspond directly with objectives. Well written multiple choice questions are appropriate to assess basic knowledge. Online examinations can be given to provide formative

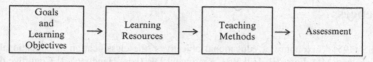

Fig. 12.1 Course design summary

feedback as well as summative assessment. As course design better embraces competency-based education, competency-aligned methods of evaluation will be necessary to assess communication skills, clinical care, and professionalism. Such methods may include direct observation, evaluations by peers, patients and other healthcare professionals, and techniques such as simulation and standardized patient interactions. Assessing the acquisition of skills such as practice-based learning and systems-based care must also be considered in the initial course design. In the past, these skills have been assessed subjectively, primarily by attending physicians and residents. Additional assessment techniques will need to be identified or developed in the future. A more comprehensive discussion of assessment follows in Chap. 15.

Summary

In summary, this chapter has discussed the principles of overall course design, emphasizing the concept of backward design: outlining what should students be able to do by the end of the course, and then determining what they must learn in order to achieve the target levels of knowledge and performance. From this specification will come the course goals and objectives, which must be consistent with the overall curricular goals and objectives. Learning resources must be identified, and the appropriate teaching methods for the course must be determined. Finally, but no less important, appropriate assessment and feedback approaches must be selected. Each of these steps will be influenced by the resources available and often by institutional policies and/or politics. While these guiding principles provide an overview of course design, several issues that are particularly important to medical students must be addressed by the faculty or course director. As faculty or course director, you can maximize the effectiveness of your efforts by incorporating the essential elements of effective design; carefully considering the relevant principles and methodologies; taking into account the needs of the students, the institution and the profession; and focusing your course design and methodology on the end results, the acquisition of foundational knowledge and skills, along with entry-level competency to apply the basic knowledge and skills appropriately.

References

Bloom BS (1956) Taxonomy of educational objectives: the classification of educational goals. In: Engelhart MD, Furst EJ, Hill WH, Krathwohl DR (eds) Handbook 1: Cognitive domain. David McKay, New York

Dent JA, Harden RM (2009) A practical guide for medical teachers. Elsevier, Edinburgh

Gage NL (1972) Teacher effectiveness and teacher education. Pacific Books, Palo Alto

Kern DE, Thomas PA, Howard DM, Bass EB (1998) Curriculum development for medical education: a six-step approach. The Johns Hopkins Press, Baltimore, pp 28–32

Knowles MS, Holton EF III, Swanson RA (1973) The adult learner: the definitive class in adult education and human resource development, 5th edn. Gulf Publishing Co, Houston

Mager RF (1962) Preparing instructional objectives: a critical tool in the development of effective instruction, 3rd edn. The Center for Effective Performance, Inc, Atlanta, pp 3–10

Mann KV (1999) Motivation in medical education: how theory can inform our practice. Acad Med 74(3):237–239

Svinicki M (1993–1994) What they don't know can hurt them: the role of prior knowledge in learning. Teaching Excellence. Prof Organ Dev Netw Higher Educ 5(4):1–2

Wiggins GP, McTighe J (2005) Chapter 1. Backward design (trans: McTighe J) Understanding by design, Expanded 2nd edn. Association for Supervision and Curriculum Development, Alexandria, pp 13–34

Chapter 13
Establishing and Teaching Elective Courses

Michele P. Pugnaire and Melissa A. Fischer

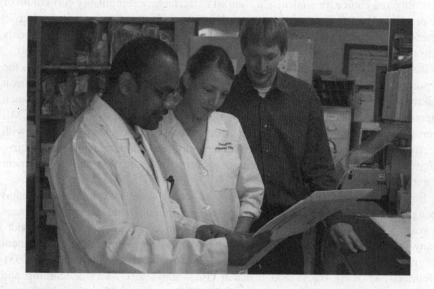

Abstract Electives have long been an integral and well-established component of medical educational programs in the United States. Beyond the year 4 electives traditionally targeted at career exploration, there has been growing interest in electives designed for enrichment and in elective experiences in years 1 through 3. This chapter provides an opportunity to consider electives in medical education as an important and often under-recognized component of the required curriculum.

M.P. Pugnaire, M.D. (✉)
University of Massachusetts Medical School,
55 Lake Avenue North, S1-119, Worcester, MA 01655, USA

M.A. Fischer, M.D., M.Ed.
University of Massachusetts School of Medicine, Worcester, MA, USA

K.N. Huggett and W.B. Jeffries (eds.), *An Introduction to Medical Teaching*,
DOI 10.1007/978-94-017-9066-6_13, © Springer Science+Business Media Dordrecht 2014

Background and Overview

Electives have long been an integral and well-established component of medical educational programs in the United States. The general purpose of electives in medical schools has been clearly articulated by accreditation standards set forth by the LCME (2012) which requires electives as a required part of the education program, serving three broad aims:

- To supplement other required courses and clerkships
- To permit career exploration through exposure to diverse medical specialties
- To provide enrichment opportunity through the pursuit of individual academic interests.

Traditionally focused on the fourth or final year of study, electives have provided flexibility and choice for students, in contrast to the largely compulsory curriculum of the preclinical and clerkship years. In year 4, trends are favoring an increase in elective time; this represents a departure from a relatively stable baseline in the prior 20 years ranging from 22.3 to 23.3 weeks from 1988 to 2009 (Barzansky and Etzel 2009).

Reports by others (Walling and Merando 2010; Slavin et al. 2003) support the importance of academic advising and guidance in elective choice and decision making, to ensure the quality of elective experiences for students. The need for such oversight as part of elective programs in medical school is clearly stated in LCME accreditation standards that require an effective system for assisting students with elective choice. Other administrative requirements and challenges include elective program approval, student assessment, programmatic evaluation and management of extramural electives.

Beyond the year 4 electives traditionally targeted at career exploration, there has been growing interest in electives designed for enrichment and in elective experiences in years 1 through 3. Fueled by the recent call for curriculum reform nationwide, many medical schools are now redesigning elective opportunities to complement programmatic innovations such as longitudinal pathways (Slavin et al. 2003), integrated scholarly tracks and research (Frishman 2001), service-learning and global health programs (Thompson et al. 2003; Dowell and Merrylees 2009); and electives designed to address specific areas of identified curricular need, such as complementary and alternative medicine (Wetzel et al. 1998), student wellness (Lee and Graham 2001), and the medical humanities (Shapiro et al. 2004).

Given the trends in the overall increase in elective time, the expansion of electives across all 4 years, the growing diversity of electives, and their integration into the redesign of curricular programs, a "nuts and bolts" review of electives in contemporary medical education is both timely and relevant. This chapter will provide this overview in three sections:

- The educational context of electives (purpose, types, methods, and models)
- Operationalizing electives (assessment, evaluation, oversight, accreditation requirements)
- Best practices and challenges (with exemplars and novel approaches)

Purpose, Definitions and Methodology

Given the evolving trends of innovation and change in medical education, the scope and breadth of electives have flourished in recent years. In many ways, electives remain a close link to the apprenticeship model of medical education which was predominant in pre-Flexner years (Ludmerer 1999). In the post-Flexner framework of traditional core education with layered electives, however, they have become an even richer asset to medical students and our healthcare system.

Electives can be divided into categories based on timing, length, sponsor or objective. A review of the medical literature reveals a variety of purposes for electives, that can be summarized in eight general categories as follows, with each described in greater detail:

1. Educational enrichment
2. Traditional medical career or "specialty" exploration
3. Complementary career exploration
4. "Audition" rotation
5. Educational remediation or support
6. Filling curricular gaps or "orphan" topics
7. Self-designed
8. Quality of life

Educational Enrichment

Students complete an educational enrichment elective in order to enhance their knowledge, skills or attitudes in order to better prepare them for entry into supervised practice. Examples of those to enhance knowledge include those that are not directly related to their field of choice. For example, national organizations may recommend that students complete specific high yield electives to "continue the acquisition of a broad base of general medical knowledge and skills" that complement career choice (Walton et al. 1993; Hull 1978). These include electives to build knowledge in areas as diverse as intensive care, dermatology, care of the elderly and radiology. With regards to skills, students may choose electives that either build discipline-specific skills such as surgical techniques to better prepare them for internship (Debas at al. 2005), or they may select courses that prepare them more generally through dedicated practice in skills of interviewing (Ang 2002) or physical exam. These electives often utilize experiential learning techniques including simulation, task trainers, trigger videos and standardized patients. Finally some educational enrichment electives focus on helping students develop competence in attitudinal areas such as empathy (Shapiro et al. 2004) or spirituality (Ousager and Johannessen 2010). Such electives can be broad in scope, engaging the arts and humanities (Ousager and Johannessen 2010) in teaching.

Medical Career Exploration

The expanding number of ACGME accredited specialties and subspecialties, that have increased nearly three-fold from 36 in 1980 to 103 in 2000 (Donini-Lenhoff and Hedrick 2000), has fueled the role of electives in medical care exploration and decision making. In light of this rapid growth of specialty career options, students who are not decided in their career plans approach the final year of medical school with the need to explore career options through elective experiences. This may be because their exposure to disciplines beyond the core clerkships has been limited, because of broad interests, or because many fields remain appealing to them at this stage of their learning. These students tend to use electives for career exploration or to solidify their interests (Walton et al. 1993). They may complete electives in traditional areas such as medical or surgical subspecialties, or those that are newer or occupy little time in the core clerkship experiences, areas such as hospice (Ousager and Johannessen 2010) or prevention (Slavin et al. 2003; Eckhert et al. 2000).

Complementary Career Exploration

In addition to medical career exploration, a growing number of electives are being established to provide educational opportunities for students in areas that provide complementary career development outside of a traditional medical field. These may include more generalizable skills such as research (Herold et al. 2002; Frishman 2001), teaching (Pasquale and Pugnaire 2002), leadership (Moseley et al. 2002), or those that are more specifically applicable such as training in International Medical Education (Thompson et al. 2003).

Audition Rotation

In the 1980s senior students began to complete more electives in their specific field of interest with a primary goal not of building skills or solidifying their choice of career, but to audition at a specific residency site where they were interested in continuing training. Identified as the "preresidency syndrome" (Swanson 1985) this practice continues today with many students completing multiple similar rotations at a number of different hospitals in order to learn about the local training culture and to demonstrate their own skills (Walton et al. 1993; Slavin et al. 2003).

Educational Remediation or Support

A number of electives are designed to address student deficiencies or help develop their learning skills and promote ongoing academic achievement. These can be classified as remediation electives, which may be tailored to student need such as clinical skills with a focus on a student's specific needs such as problem-solving or physical examination competence. They can also address broader areas which will be applicable in the future such as time management, dealing with uncomfortable situations or promoting lifelong learning (Cheever et al. 2002).

Filling Curricular Gaps or "Orphan" Topics

A growing body of medical science knowledge and ongoing expansion of fields of practice dictates the need for electives that fill gaps in the curriculum. Such electives cover so-called orphan topics which do not readily find a home in core teaching. This may be because they span multiple disciplines or because they are truly niche areas which are important for study in a limited number of fields. Such electives include topics such as complementary and alternative medicine (Wetzel et al. 1998), pain management (Puljak and Sapunar 2011) and palliative care (Weissman and Griffie 1998). These electives can stand alone, or be integrated to create a multi-dimensional program. For instance a series of electives described to teach about pain include "The Puzzle of Pain" focusing on neurobiology and basic science concepts, "Empathy and Pain" which uses humanities to teach about the emotions of pain, and "The Cochrane Library and Pain" which uses the literature related to pain management to teach evidence-based medicine skills and practice (Puljak and Sapunar 2011).

Self-Designed

Despite constant curricular adjustments based on changes in medical knowledge (Ludmerer 1999), and the availability of electives that address curricular gaps as noted above, students continue to identify topics of interest which are not included in the core curriculum or existing electives. These needs can be filled by self-designed electives which students can customize to their own needs. Sometimes called an independent study, this type of elective can be clinical or not, and must still meet LCME accreditation requirements for credit. Generally students must complete an application that includes specific information regarding objectives, activities and time commitment, as well as identifying a faculty sponsor who will be responsible for any necessary assessment and grading.

Quality of Life

This sort of elective can fall into several categories, and thus may not warrant its own heading, however it is important to recognize that sometimes students take electives to improve their short or long-term quality of life. With respect to short-term some students take specific electives which they perceive as less-rigorous in order to provide respite between the intensity of clerkships and internship, or to allow for residency interviews. Those that may have longer-term benefits include electives that teach skills that support quality of life such as time management or wellness (Lee and Graham 2001) and may be pre-existing or self-designed.

Electives vs. Selectives

For the purposes of this chapter we use the definitions from our own student handbook which describes the term elective as "a structured learning experience in a field of medicine or related fields approved by the faculty … which is not specifically required as part of the basic medical school curriculum." (UMMS student handbook: http://www.umassmed.edu/studentaffairs/electiveprogram.aspx, Accessed 4/22/13). LCME accredited medical schools must define the number of elective weeks available to students, how many elective credits must be completed and any requirements regarding the area or categorization of electives (see section on operationalizing below regarding current requirements). As such, electives provide the primary means for students to personalize or add flexibility to their medical education. While similar in that they support student choice for individual study, "selectives" are generally a smaller number of scheduled activities from which a student must choose a certain number as part of their graduation requirements. For example, Herold et al. (2002) describe a selective program at Mount Sinai School of Medicine which required students to select either a research or one of six disease-focused cores thus allowing for limited choice to meet a requirement.

While required by the LCME to offer electives, programs maintain substantial choice in their structure and function. In addition to the categories of electives described above, US medical schools have developed elective programs that can occur during all years in student learning, are time-limited or longitudinal, are graded or simply recorded for credit. Further details regarding innovations and best practices are described below and support the creative elective models that have been designed to meet the needs of students, faculty and educational programs.

Operationalizing Electives in Medical Schools

Given the flexibility, variety, and diverse purposes of electives in medical schools, administrative systems must be in place to assure the successful implementation, consistency and educational quality of elective experiences. Such oversight of electives must be formally established in medical schools, given the LCME accreditation standards that specify the roles and responsibilities required for meeting compliance with the institutional oversight of electives. This oversight typically resides in the office of student affairs, given the pre-eminent role of electives in career exploration, residency preparation and in addressing a variety of individual student needs. Not surprisingly, the LCME standards for electives are housed in both the "Medical Student" section of the LCME standards, pertaining to elective management and oversight, as well as in "Educational Program for the MD Degree" standards, which focuses on requirements pertaining to electives as part of the overall curriculum.

The accreditation requirements pertaining to electives do not specify criteria for duration (i.e., number for weeks or months); scheduling within particular components in the curriculum; specific content, educational methodology or pedagogy; or required topics or specialty areas that must be represented in elective offerings. To the contrary, programmatic requirements for electives are comparatively modest, in contrast to depth and breadth of standards that apply to the "required" preclinical and clinical courses and clerkships. This permits a relatively broad range of accredited elective opportunities to be managed and overseen by offices for student affairs. As with all accredited curricular programs, electives must be institutionally sponsored by a suitable department or office, and authorized by the school to grant academic credit for an educational program. Most typically, electives are departmentally sponsored, but may also have sponsorship conferred by other official school entities such as an office of medical education or an office for research, for example. As well, extramural electives that are sponsored by entities outside the organization may be recognized for "elective credit" by a medical school, providing that there is a system in place for assuring that the extramural experience meets the equivalency for an elective at the home institution. The AAMC provides resources such as the Extramural Electives Compendium data base and VSAS (the visiting student application service) to promote accessibility to and scheduling of approved accredited extramural electives at LCME-accredited medical schools nationwide.

At the level of institutional oversight for management of intramural electives, accreditation standards require that "electives permit medical students to gain exposure to and deepen their understanding of medical specialties reflecting their career interests" as well as "provide opportunities for medical students to pursue individual academic interests." In keeping with this standard, the LCME currently requires medical schools undergoing accreditation to report the following information regarding accredited electives (LCME 2013):

- The number of weeks of elective time that are expected of all medical students in each year of the curriculum.
- The maximum number of weeks that students may spend taking electives at another institution that is not part of the medical school's health system or affiliated with the medical school.
- The average number of weeks that students in the most recent graduating class spent taking electives at another institution.
- Description of any policies or practices that encourage students to use electives to pursue interests outside of their chosen specialty.
- Indicate any policies in place that specify a maximum number of electives (or elective weeks) that a given student may take in the same specialty area, either at the home medical school or extramurally.

To a certain extent, these standards serve to mitigate the concerns about electives that are commonly cited in the ongoing debate about the merits and limitations of the fourth year of the educational program. These concerns include:

- Relative lack of consistency and comparability across the diversity of elective experiences (Slavin et al. 2003; Walling and Merando 2010)
- The perceived limitations of rigor in assessment (Slavin et al. 2003)
- The inconsistency of motivation and purpose for student elective choice, ranging from "audition electives" to self-designed electives (Walling and Merando 2010)
- The inherent limitations of assuring the equivalency of elective credit, rigor and value, particularly given the diversity of accredited elective formats, ranging from 1 week (Pasquale and Pugnaire 2002) to 2 months or more (Imperato 2004; Frishman 2001)

Given the above concerns, and the pros and cons of electives discussed previously, a successful elective program must provide quality guidance and consistent oversight to students, in the selection and institutional approval of their preferred elective experiences. Reinforcing this need, the LCME accreditation standards require effective systems for assisting medical students in choosing elective courses. For example, for those medical schools undergoing accreditation in 2012–2013, the LCME requested the following information regarding student guidance and oversight in choice of electives:

- Identification of the individual(s) primarily responsible for providing guidance to medical students about their intramural and extramural elective choices, across all years of the curriculum
- The role(s) or title(s) of individual(s) responsible for the formal approval of medical students' elective courses in each year of the curriculum
- Data that documents student satisfaction with guidance in the choice of electives

These accreditation standards and reporting requirements support the importance of an administrative structure for elective management and oversight that provides centralized, coordinated, comprehensive and readily accessible elective guidance to all students enrolled in accredited elective experiences.

Best Practices, Challenges and Exemplars

Given the diversity of expectations and possibilities that electives offer, it is no surprise that there are so many varieties. Electives are an ideal opportunity for students, faculty, and educational programs to develop creative and "proactive" curricular offerings that respond nimbly to the changing needs of students, educational programs, and regulatory requirements in medical education, both current and anticipated. Recognizing these unique and important features of electives, this section provides an overview of best practices and the current challenges of electives in medical education. The scope of this overview will highlight the diversity of electives that fall outside the domain of the traditional 4th year variety offered in clinical disciplines and subspecialty rotations. These "traditional year 4 electives" generally follow a similar structure and administrative management as the traditional, core clinical clerkships. As part of this focus on the broader range of electives, three exemplars of contemporary elective innovations will be described, showcasing the wide spectrum of electives that are evolving in diverse content areas across all 4 years of the educational program. These three novel, non-traditional elective structures will address distinct, thematic innovations, to illustrate the variety and adaptability of electives.

Best Practices and Challenges

Some common challenges shared by electives of all types include: enrollment, student assessment, program evaluation and faculty development. While these challenges can also be encountered in required curricula, the diversity of sites, expectations, structure, and number of faculty involved add unique complexity to the challenges encountered in developing and administering elective courses and clinical rotations. As previously described, in order to ensure optimal educational value for students' elective experience, formal guidance is needed in choosing electives and assisting students in developing their personal educational plan (PEP) for elective experiences. This plan must be appropriately time-framed to conform to elective enrollment periods, inform elective sponsors about the enrollment roster, and to verify that all graduation requirements are fulfilled. In addition, specific rules regarding timing and process for changing the PEP are critical. If students can disenroll close to the start of an elective, faculty may become disillusioned and refuse future students. In contrast, if students add new electives too close to the start faculty may not be prepared to accept them on a rotation. In addition, changes late in a cycle may compromise students' readiness for graduation.

Faculty advisors should receive specific training in order to understand the breadth and depth of elective opportunities, evaluate student need, meet school graduation requirements and incorporate any residency application implications into student choice. A common practice is to assign students one on one with a designated faculty advisor for such guidance. In the best of these pairings the student will benefit from direct personal mentoring, advising, and faculty expertise. Common limitations of such arrangements include difficulty in scheduling meetings, variability in the effectiveness and quality of counseling, and the potential for missing opportunities and deadlines. Some medical schools have established more rigorous programs for supporting students' elective planning and advising needs. These programs may include academies of teachers, mentors, or learning communities that are designed to provide more consistent and higher quality advising by supporting a smaller number of better prepared faculty (Ferguson et al. 2009). While these programs have many potential benefits, they may be more resource intensive to establish and maintain.

Student assessment in elective programs is based largely on faculty observation of performance, with comparatively less effort devoted to more objective measures generally obtained through written tests or demonstration of skills through simulated or standardized patient experiences. Fair and reliable assessment in such circumstances is complicated by the large number of faculty who may participate in elective teaching at irregular intervals. The discontinuity of faculty participation presents a particular challenge for ensuring appropriate orientation to the elective experience as well as the timely, accurate and consistent completion of student performance assessments. Faculty participating in electives who are responsible for student assessment should receive basic training and clear guidelines regarding such performance standards and expectations. It is helpful to use consistent, standardized evaluation forms for measuring programmatic quality and learner performance across electives. Core items should also be included on programmatic evaluations for electives to support individual quality improvement and program development by allowing comparisons of quality measures across diverse elective experiences. Even with well-designed assessment and evaluation forms, and faculty development, collecting completed forms from faculty and students is often more challenging in electives than for required rotations. This again reflects the large number of students and faculty participating, as well as the dispersed and diverse locations for elective programs, and the fact that students may spend anywhere from 1 week to 3 years, in an elective experience. The management of elective evaluations thus requires robust and well-coordinated administrative support to process the large the number of evaluations that must be completed and tracked. As well, schools must determine how to weigh the relative credits allocated to individual electives, across a wide range of diverse elective experiences, with some as short as 1-week and others lasting years. A centralized school office, commonly under the oversight of the dean for student affairs, is typically charged with overseeing elective enrollment, performance assessment and grade submission; student elective advising and approval; monitoring quality across elective programs; and maintaining current and complete rosters of elective offerings. In addition, this office is likely to contribute to ongoing efforts to review and revise elective practices to best meet the challenges of elective programs and the needs of students.

Exemplars of Innovation

To best illustrate the diversity, creativity and adaptability of electives in meeting a variety of needs in contemporary educational programs, three novel, non-traditional electives will be described. These have been selected to represent a variety of innovations, with each elective representing a distinct methodological theme as noted below:

- Brief core clinical year experience http://www.umassmed.edu/FCE.aspx?linkide ntifier=id&itemid=144682

- Non-accredited, multi-year electives http://www.umassmed.edu/UME/OEE.aspx
- Competitive Longitudinal Professional Development Pathways http://www.umassmed.edu/oume/rso/ctrp.aspx

Brief Core Clinical Year Experience

Housed in the core clinical year or the traditional 3rd year of the curriculum, a model of "Flexible Clinical Experiences" or FCE's has been established at UMass Medical School (UMMS). The FCE's are brief, 1 or 2-week, accredited elective experiences designed to expand more traditional elective opportunities and support students' exploration of a variety of clinical and translational science fields, early in their education (as early as June of the 2nd academic year). The FCE program allows for one month of total FCE experience in the course of the core clinical clerkship rotations. The FCE program supports self-directed learning by allowing students to either choose from a diverse offering of pre-designed electives or to create their own experience. The advantages of early exposure to a medical specialty include the opportunity to foster mentorships, nurture and develop interests in a specialty, supplement learning in areas related to their field of choice or those not covered in the core curriculum and to allow brief episodes of career exploration that can help students determine whether to devote more time during traditional 4th year elective periods. In addition, students requiring remediation may apply to use limited FCE time, and those presenting their work at society conferences can apply for a self-designed FCE in order to receive credit for conference attendance and presentation. In the interest of avoiding the "preresidency syndrome," students complete a minimum of three distinct experiences, and the experiences are in at least two different departments within or outside the medical school.

Non-accredited, Multi-year Electives

This non-accredited, interprofessional multi-year longitudinal elective model, the Optional Enrichment Elective (OEE), was designed to provide students with low stakes opportunities for exploring non-core curricula at times that meet their needs. These elective courses are offered in addition to the regular, required and elective/selective curriculum, and as such are unlike regular electives in that the student may choose to not take any of them. They are scheduled during the "independent study" or other unscheduled time in the curriculum calendar (often afternoons, evenings, weekends or during "protected time.") Participation in these courses is mentioned in the dean's letter and appears on the transcript by name of course, but there is no grade associated. Failure to complete course requirements results simply in the course not being listed on the student's transcript. It is not possible to "fail" such a course.

The UMass Medical School Optional Enrichment Electives are longitudinal experiences of varying lengths lasting at least 1 semester. They can only be proposed by students and thus are designed to best meet student needs, though they must have a faculty sponsor, and must be approved by the educational policy committee which is the curricular governing body of the school. Current topics include: Adoption and Foster Care, Navigator Program in Geriatrics, Students as Educators, Roads to Recovery: Substance Abuse from Patients' Perspective, Wilderness Medicine and Recreational Emergencies, Medical Creative Writing and American Sign Language.

Competitive Longitudinal Professional Development Pathway

While the electives described above are open to all students as space allows, some electives require application and students are selected to participate. At UMMS these include longitudinal elective experiences in Global Health, Care of Rural and Underserved Patients, and a Clinical and Translational Research Pathway (CTRP). Designed to serve students willing to make a longer term commitment to following a longitudinal parallel medical school curriculum and develop targeted professional skills, these programs require substantial student and institutional commitments. Students in these pathways attain increased competence in the areas of focus through dedicated extra-curricular activities that include didactics, mentorship, experiential learning and public presentation of scholarly work. Participation in such programs can prepare students to assume higher level responsibilities in residency and beyond. In some core medical school classes, CTRP students are grouped together for optimal coordination with the traditional curriculum. Successful participation culminates in receipt of a "Certificate of Training in Clinical/Translational Research," notation on the transcript and MSPE but no formal grade, nor do these Pathways fulfill any graduation requirements.

Summary

In closing, this overview has provided an opportunity to consider electives in medical education as an important and often under-recognized component of the required curriculum. The flexibility, adaptability and diversity of elective formats has fueled the growth of elective offerings and expanded the representation of elective opportunities across all 4 years of the educational program. Current challenges in the administration of electives focus on the need for timely, consistent and high quality advising to assist students with planning and approving electives selections. With the ever expanding demand for new content in medical school curricula and the diversity of elective models under development in our medical schools nationwide, elective programs will continue to thrive and provide important educational value to our students and to medical education. This is perhaps best summarized in the comments of a former student at the University of Massachusetts Medical School who wrote "[electives provided some of] my favorite experiences in medical school.

The attendings and the residents were excellent teachers. I saw amazing cases and always felt part of the team. Exposure to the field through this unique, wonderful group of people is what made me want to go into ..."

References

Ang M (2002) Advanced communication skills: conflict management and persuasion. Acad Med 77:1166

Barzansky B, Etzel S (2009) Medical schools in the United States, 2008–2009. JAMA 302:1349–1355

Cheever T, Norman C, Nora L (2002) Improving medical students' comfort with, and skill in handling gender-related inquiries during the residency selection process. Acad Med 77:11

Debas HT, Bass BL, Brennan MF et al (2005) American Surgical Association Blue Ribbon Committee Report on Surgical Education: 2004. Ann Surg 241:1–8

Donini-Lenhoff FG, Hedrick HL (2000) Growth of specialization in graduate medical education. JAMA 284:1284–1289

Dowell J, Merrylees N (2009) Electives: isn't it time for a change? Med Educ 43:121–126

Eckhert NL, Bennett NM, Grande D, Dandoy S (2000) Teaching prevention through electives. Acad Med 75(7 Suppl):S85–S89

Ferguson KJ, Wolter EM, Yarbrough DB, Carline JD, Krupat E (2009) Defining and describing medical learning communities: results of a national survey. Acad Med 84:1549–1556

Frishman WH (2001) Student research projects and theses: should they be a requirement for medical school graduation? Heart Dis 3:141–144

Herold B, McArdle P, Stagnaro-Green A (2002) Translational medicine in the first year: integrative cores. Acad Med 77(11):1171

Hull DS (1978) Elective subjects for medical students preparing for a career in ophthalmology. Ophthalmology 85:12

Imperato PJ (2004) A Third World international health elective for U.S. medical students: the 25-year experience of the State University of New York, Downstate Medical Center. J Commun Health 29:337–373

Lee J, Graham AV (2001) Students' perception of medical school stress and their evaluation of a wellness elective. Med Educ 35:652–659

Liaison Committee on Medical Education (2012) Accreditation standards. Revised June 2013. http://www.lcme.org/publications/functions2013june.pdf. Accessed 4 Dec 2013

Liaison Committee on Medical Education (2013) Data collection instrument – Full Accreditation Visit. http://www.lcme.org/survey-connect-dci-download.htm. Accessed 4 Dec 2013

Ludmerer KM (1999) Time to heal: American medical education from the turn of the century to the era of managed care. Oxford University Press, New York

Moseley T, Cantrell M, Deloney L (2002) Clinical skills center attending: an innovative senior medical school elective. Acad Med 77:1176

Ousager J, Johannessen H (2010) Humanities in undergraduate medical education: a literature review. Acad Med 85:988–998

Pasquale SJ, Pugnaire MP (2002) Preparing medical students to teach. Acad Med 77:1175–1176

Puljak L, Sapunar D (2011) Web-Based elective courses for medical students: an example in pain. Pain Med 12:854–863

Shapiro J, Morrison EH, Boker JR (2004) Teaching empathy to first year medical students: evaluation of an elective literature and medicine course. Educ Health 17:73–84

Slavin S, Wilkes M, Ussatine R, Hoffman J (2003) Curricular reform of the 4th year of medical school: The Colleges Model. Teach Learn Med 15:183–193

Swanson AG (1985) The 'Preresidency Syndrome': an incipient epidemic of educational disruption. J Med Educ 60:201–202

Thompson MJ, Huntington MK, Hunt DD, Pinsky LE, Brodie JJ (2003) Educational effects of International Health Electives on U.S. and Canadian Medical Students and Residents: a literature review. Acad Med 78:342–347

Walling A, Merando A (2010) The fourth year of medical school: a literature review. Acad Med 85:1698–1704

Walton LA, Fenner DE, Seltzer VL, Wilbanks GD, Laube DW, Crenshaw MC, Messer RH, Hale RH (1993) The fourth-year medical school curriculum: recommendations of the Association of Professors of Gynecology and Obstetrics and the Council on Resident Education in Obstetrics and Gynecology. Am J Obstet Gynecol 169:13–16

Weissman DE, Griffie J (1998) Integration of palliative medicine at the Medical College of Wisconsin, 1990–1996. J Pain Symp Manage 15:195–201

Wetzel MS, Eisenberg DM, Kaptchuk TJ (1998) Courses involving Complementary and Alternative Medicine at US Medical Schools. JAMA 280:784–787. doi:10.1001/jama.280.9.784. http://jama.jamanetwork.com/article.aspx?articleid=187927

Chapter 14
Designing Global Health Experiences

Katrin Sara Sadigh, David Chia, and Majid Sadigh

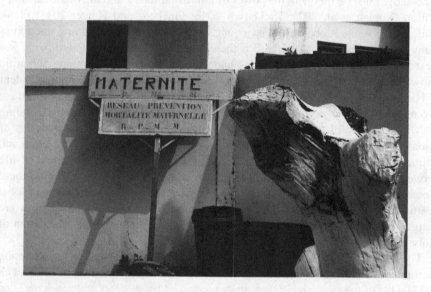

Abstract Enthusiasm around global health is burgeoning across medical institutions. More students are entering the field of medicine versed in the language of global health and equipped to take on roles with social and humanistic dimensions. They look to institutional administrators to not only provide them with avenues to engage this interest, but to exemplify the goals and vision of the global health movement.

K.S. Sadigh, M.D. (✉) • D. Chia, M.D., M.Sc.
Yale Internal Medicine Primary Care Residency Program, New Haven, CT, USA
e-mail: katrin.sadigh@yale.edu

M. Sadigh, M.D.
Danbury Hospital/Western Connecticut Health Center, University of Vermont College
of Medicine, Burlington, VT, USA

K.N. Huggett and W.B. Jeffries (eds.), *An Introduction to Medical Teaching*,
DOI 10.1007/978-94-017-9066-6_14, © Springer Science+Business Media Dordrecht 2014

In the face of this momentous expectation, program leadership has an opportunity to guide the next generation of citizens of the world: individuals who will become leaders in global health, creators of scientific knowledge, and instruments of change in the dispelling of disparities.

Why Global Health?

Global health is collaborative transnational research and action for promoting health for all (Beaglehole and Bonita 2010). It endeavors to improve health and quality of life through the prevention and control of disease, injury, and disability while taking into account the complex socioeconomic, political, and cultural determinants that necessarily must be met with the power of interdisciplinary and international cooperation (Koplan et al. 2009; Kickbusch 2006; Fineberg and Hunter 2013; Frenk et al. 2010). While global health as a concept has been steadily gaining traction in many different sectors of society, it is the escalating abject poverty worldwide and increasing disparities in health status and care in the face of booming scientific knowledge that instills a sense of urgency. Lawrence Summers, the former president of Harvard University, speaks of the great weight to be borne by both: "There are two major issues the world must address in the next 30 years. One is the expanding knowledge of the life sciences, which promises understanding of mechanisms of disease, of means to prevent and treat disease, and of functioning of the brain and ultimately the mind. The second is the increasing disparities in quality of life between and within countries. Global Health stands as the fulcrum linking these global agendas." Thus, the role to be played by universities in establishing global health programs is clear: as the seat of creation of knowledge, universities are obliged to take on the role of applying this knowledge towards the eradication of global disparities.

The lessons learned and skills gained for medical students and residents during their international experiences are multifold and cannot be overstated (Wilson et al. 2012). One of the most significant attributes gained by students and residents is an understanding of the multifaceted influence of culture on the healthcare delivery and outcomes (Garfunkel and Howard 2011). Not only are students and residents able to dismantle the absolutist notions of "right" versus "wrong," but also they are better able to appreciate the complexities posed by culture on medical belief systems (Mao et al. 2007). Additionally, students and residents become better equipped to recognize and manage tropical and infectious diseases, a vital skill in light of globalization, immigration and international travel. Where resources such as advanced imaging modalities and litanies of laboratory tests are scarce, students and residents are challenged to adapt, to hone their diagnostic skills and to refine their powers of observation. Many studies have shown that students and residents who have had international experiences subsequently are less reliant on diagnostic testing, have broader differential diagnoses and exhibit greater adeptness with the physical exam (Drain et al. 2007). Moreover, students and residents who have had international experiences are more likely to have careers working with underserved populations both domestically and abroad. One study demonstrated that 57 % of medical students went on to commit time to another resource-limited country, 67 % to community health projects, and another 31 % spending the majority of their time working with the underserved (Ramsey et al. 2004). Another manner in which global health experiences shape the career path of medical students is their greater commitment to primary care and public health: in this same study, 74 % pursued primary care residency training compared to 45 % of all US medical graduates, 29 % pursued a Master in Public Health (MPH) compared to 3 % (Ramsey et al. 2004). The resultant increased capacity for cultural competence and communication, as well as an enhanced sense of the importance of the interface between medicine, public health and primary care, are not only essential in the international setting, but also equip medical students to more effectively respond to the ever rising health disparities and diversity in patient populations in the United States. Medical students gain insight into themselves and others as they are challenged to redefine their relationship with people and environments, acquire maturity and learn humility, attributes desired by residency programs and the profession itself (Smith and Weaver 2006).

The Association of American Medical Colleges (AAMC) reports a rise in the number of graduating medical students who took part in a global health experience from 6 % in 1984 to 25 % in 2004 (AAMC 2012). Currently, applicants to medical school and residency programs increasingly ask about international programs and more than half factor it into their decision (Garfunkel and Howard 2011). This interest in pursuing a career in global health often begins before students apply to medical school. Indeed, the promise of medicine as a vehicle for change and alleviation of suffering has not been dispelled for many students. They are catalyzed by a genuine interest in social justice and a sense of responsibility for global stewardship. Others may be led by a scientific curiosity in infectious diseases and the underserved populations they often afflict, or by an interest in public health and health policy. Given the growing role played by the media in depicting worldwide events and bringing personal and national narratives to light in greater detail, the desire of individuals to make their personal contributions begins to take shape earlier. By the time students begin medical school, many not only have a great interest in global health, but they are asking pointed questions about the capacity of medical school programs to provide necessary resources. Students who do not begin medical school with this interest in global health are often led towards the field by the enthusiasm expressed by their classmates and by the disparities they are confronted with as they care for patients from immigrant, refugee, and marginalized populations. These students begin to understand that the concepts of global health are not confined to the international health arena. Instead, they come to realize that in order to deliver more meaningful and sustainable care to their patients here in the United States, they must become better versed in subjects exploring the underlying discrepancies in access to healthcare.

In spite of the growing demand among students for substantive international experiences in medical school and residency, opportunities for them to enroll in an organized global health curriculum are limited (Peluso et al. 2013). Medical schools and universities can play a pivotal role in global health by identifying promising students, cultivating their interest and promoting their growth into global citizens. These institutions can then lead efforts to unite both nationally and internationally with a shared agenda to build educational, research, and clinical programs centered on unified goals of healthcare and social equity. Most global health programs begin by initially offering classes in global health and tropical medicine as well as presentations and events as part of student interest groups. Students subsequently become involved in organizing community health fairs and rotating through immigrant, refugee and travel clinics. While these aforementioned opportunities are offered by the majority of medical schools and provide a good starting point, establishing mature academic relationships with resource-limited communities, both urban and rural, national and international, should be the ultimate vision and allows for a more robust and authentic curriculum and partnership (Francis et al. 2012; Frenk et al. 2010). It is the hope that participants of such a program will be stirred in profound ways that will inspire some into leadership positions in the field of global health, thereby creating the cascade of knowledge and capacity building necessary to tackle the disparities in health and society.

Before setting down the principles and details involved in the initiation of a global health program, it is important to depict its general shape. Specifically, one must envision two sister institutions: the first within the United States and the second at an international site. Each institution must be equipped with a clear understanding of its roles as well as the resources with which each shall carry out its roles. The fundamental premise of academic collaborations at the international level is that both institutions share a common vision with each possessing a unique set of attributes to contribute towards this end (Crump and Sugarman 2010; Peluso et al. 2012). This notion of bi-directionality binds both parties to a relationship based on mutual respect and equal exchange. Only in this manner can both partners take ownership of their accomplishments and move forward in such a way that is enriching and self-sustaining.

The benefits inherent to international partnerships exceed that of a mere exchange. Indeed, when done successfully, these partnerships are presented with the opportunity to become more than they can be individually (Drain et al. 2007). Theoretical concepts pertaining to disease and epidemics become a truer reality formed from the on-the-ground experiences both parties share, while each offering their own unique vantage point based on their historical and sociocultural narratives. This ebb and flow allows for the rapid exchange of knowledge, the creation of novel solutions, and the flourishing of a culture of learning that is spared the destruction of transplantation when they are allowed to be adopted with patience. As a more rigorous academic atmosphere is fostered and prescribed notions of healthcare delivery are challenged, hope builds towards improved patient outcomes (Balandin et al. 2007; Drain et al. 2007).

One particularly promising shared goal is capacity building through investment in human resources. For instance, several institutions have developed exchanges whereby physicians from resource-limited settings are given the opportunity to pursue advanced training, often difficult to acquire in their own countries, at sponsoring academic medical centers (Crump and Sugarman 2010; Garfunkel and Howard 2011; Rabin and Schwartz 2012). Candidates are chosen based on their potential to become future leaders within the field of medicine and their commitment to improving medical education and patient care in their home country. The goal of this training would be to impart important skill sets that are currently absent in the physicians' native environment. This may involve research methodology, medical subspecialty training, and technical training (such as ultrasound-guided biopsies and echocardiography). These physicians can also be paired with a mentor at the sponsoring medical center that may lead into a lifelong academic relationship that facilitates future exchanges in a constructive cycle (Nakanjako et al. 2011). Ultimately, these individuals will become a vital segment of the leadership for the medical education system at their home institutions.

Initiation of a Global Health Program

The energy to begin and to fuel a global health program should be sought in the student body. Not only is student involvement in all aspects of program development paramount to the sustainability of the program, but also because it often takes student commitment to engage the administration and to catalyze the initiation of a global health program (Francis et al. 2012).

Regardless of whether or not a global health program exists at one's institution, inevitably there exists individuals both within the faculty, residents and student body who have meaningful global health experiences and established international connections. Therefore, an inventory of all parties should be created detailing project specifics and willingness to participate in global health courses as teachers or to serve as mentors for interested students (Francis et al. 2012).

Next, the creation and mobilization of a global health interest group not only provides a forum for already interested students to foster their interests, but also garners the engagement of students less familiar with the field (Castillo et al. 2012; Francis et al. 2012). These groups are often led by second-year medical students with membership from all four classes. A faculty member who has proven to be supportive and resourceful should be designated as their advisor. Students should lead all efforts of the interest group, including delineation of yearly objectives and organization of events and meetings. Students should be encouraged to articulate their thoughts, concerns and requests so that the goals and future direction of the group are clear. A few examples of potential projects for these interest groups include: connecting students to faculty for mentorship; establishment of tropical medicine and global health electives to supplement the medical education curriculum; organization of lecture series, journal club, and panel discussions featuring local and national student and faculty leaders. Additionally, a Global Health Day may be established that is committed to raising community awareness regarding global health topics and to showcase accomplishments in the field across different disciplines and departments.

Once the student group has solidified around core objectives, it can begin to mobilize its efforts both within and beyond the university community in order to strengthen its presence and gather support from institutional leaders, alumni, and other members in order to kick start the next phase of a maturing global health program: establishment of international partnerships. The construction of a comprehensive website can also function as a great resource for global health. This site can outline activities of the group, provide links to other informative websites, books and journals, as well as to modules on medical ethics, global health, and tropical medicine, and to share brief overviews of significant global health events both locally and across the globe.

International Partnerships

Conversations regarding international collaborations often are initiated by individuals who already have an ongoing professional relationship rather than de novo. This relationship could consist of smaller scale service projects, teaching of courses and/or clinical duties that over time solidifies into a bond that gradually grows into a larger, more significant collaboration. At this point, both parties should invest time in the drafting of a "Memorandum of Understanding" (MOU) to put in words their common vision and to prioritize their objectives. While this stage requires much effort and time, sometimes on the order of months to years, the writing of the MOU itself further strengthens the relationship between the parties as each works with the other to lay down a foundation based on sustainability, mutual respect, and capacity building (Crump and Sugarman 2010).

It is recommended that a master MOU be drafted between the administrative offices of the two collaborating universities, approved by the respective legal offices and signed by the respective provost or vice chancellor. This master MOU represents a general outline of the relationship consisting of a brief description of the general purpose of the agreement and types of cooperation to take place (including education, clinical, and research initiatives). A section outlining financial arrangements should also be included along with any concluding provisions pertaining to modifications, annexes, addenda, and renewal. Once this master MOU has been signed, it serves as an umbrella agreement between the two institutions that anchors all further collaborations between individual departments. Additional MOUs should focus on the specifics of these individual departmental relationships and should be signed by the dean of the medical school as well as the chairperson of each relevant department. All MOUs should clearly define the institutional partners and consist of sections detailing the nature and scope of the collaboration, outlining mutual requirements, describing items to which each party commits, as well as general terms of the contract.

Institutions should endeavor to gradually establish a continuous 12-month presence at the international site involving members of a multidisciplinary team (Crump and Sugarman 2010). The sustained and multidisciplinary nature of the partnership serves to help consolidate and maximize leadership training opportunities, mentorship, and community health services. Towards this end, program staff (program director and support staff) for both sites should be identified and trained in both technical and cross-cultural skills. In addition, qualified faculty members should be charged with the supervision of residents and medical students at the international site (Campagna et al. 2013). This supervision extends beyond that of a traditional preceptor with oversight of clinical duties and should embody the role of a mentor who places great care into the overall well-being of students and residents as they adjust to the life and work in a new setting (Crump and Sugarman 2010). Funds must be secured in order to: fully subsidize the salaries of program staff, faculty members, and residents; establish scholarships for international participants to the US-based institution; and provide travel grants for medical student rotations (Campagna et al. 2013). Funds also will be essential for the establishment of a global health office at each site. Donations in the form of library resources, medical supplies, and diagnostic equipment may be necessary as well (Axt et al. 2013).

It is often the case that once a collaboration has been initiated, it becomes easier for other institutional partners to envision their own involvement. The momentum that builds with the establishment of an initial MOU and the early accomplishment of set goals pulls in other interested parties. It is imperative that each new partner establishes its own MOU with which to guide its educational, clinical, and/or research activities in an individualized approach.

Programming Specifics

Selection of Students and Residents for International Electives

The backbone of global health electives is made up of the students and residents who take part in these experiences. Given their vital role, the selection process must be meticulous. A committee of faculty members should be established and placed in charge of the selection process. Applicants may be asked to provide a personal statement describing their interest in global health and the specific site of the rotation as well as outlining how the experience may tie in with career goals. They may also be asked to submit letters of recommendation from faculty members and research mentors. Interviews offer an opportunity to pose questions addressing different ethical dilemmas to identify applicants with a keen sense of cultural sensitivity and to avoid those who may prove dogmatic and ethnocentric. Students and residents who make ideal candidates for global health experiences should be adaptable, motivated to address global health issues, sensitive to local priorities, and have the ability and experiences to match the expectations of the program. It is essential that they will be good representatives of their home institution and country (Crump and Sugarman 2010). The selection process should begin early in the academic year in order to allot ample time for pre-departure preparation, including general orientation activities, passports, visas, tickets, vaccinations, medical supplies, and travel insurance (Sarfaty and Arnold 2005). It is often an expectation of selected students to commit to a project upon their return, such as giving a global health lecture, devising a case-based presentation, participating in future orientation sessions or conducting a community outreach project.

Pre-departure Preparation of US Trainees

To ensure that students and residents have a successful rotation, programs must offer them comprehensive preparation prior to their departure. The main components should include a curriculum focusing on: global health and tropical medicine; health and safety; practical logistics; cultural competence and language training. Importantly, a conversation must be had with students and residents regarding ethical issues that may arise and the proper approach to handling them (Shah and Wu 2008). It should be stressed that they will undoubtedly face challenges and uncertainties, even those that cannot be anticipated. They must accept and, to a certain extent, welcome these situations as a valuable part of the experience. They should be given guidance on ways to respond that serve to dissipate rather than inflict further damage among involved parties. Attributes such as patience, tolerance, and flexibility must be stressed. Skills such as pushing oneself to greater understanding of unfamiliar practices and rejecting quick judgments should be endorsed. Participants must embrace their defined roles and reciprocate the kindness and generosity of their hosts who have welcomed them into their culture and homes. Moreover, residents must meet local medical licensing standards and all research must be approved by institutional review boards at both the home and host sites (Crump and Sugarman 2010).

Topics in Global Health and Tropical Medicine

Classroom sessions covering pertinent general global health and specific tropical medicine topics can be organized and moderated by faculty members (Nelson et al. 2012). Medical students and residents should be encouraged to take an active role in these sessions by facilitating part of the discussion or preparing a segment of the presentation. In addition, clinical case conferences utilizing a live videoconference with faculty and students between home and international institutions have been successfully implemented and provide real-time comparative discussions regarding risk factors, clinical presentation, and management of the same disease in different settings (Goldner and Bollinger 2012). Topics in global health to be considered for inclusion in the program curriculum include those that would provide a solid foundation regarding the economic and social structures that define health care and health systems as well as a global understanding of the role played by infectious and tropical disease. A lengthy but inexhaustive list of topics includes the global burden of infectious diseases, global burden of chronic diseases, impact of foundations and public-private partnerships, the World Bank, the International Monetary Fund (IMF), intellectual property and access to medicines, social disparities on health status, health considerations of vulnerable populations, reproductive and women's health, displaced populations and war, comparative health systems and human resources, emerging diseases, water safety and sanitation, neglected diseases and research, and the role of vaccinations. Training in specific tropical medicine topics would provide participants with a basic understanding of diseases afflicting patient populations. A potential list of tropical medicine topics includes amebic diseases, brucellosis, cysticercosis, filariasis, hemorrhagic fever, human immunodeficiency virus, hydatid disease, intestinal helminths, leishmaniasis, leprosy, malaria, schistosomiasis, sleeping sickness, tuberculosis, typhoid fever, and yellow fever. Inclusion of practical skills sessions that would be useful and necessary in resource-limited settings should also be considered, including tropical microscopy, basic bedside ultrasound, simple dental extraction, splinting and wound management (Nelson et al. 2012).

Health and Safety

Students and residents should be evaluated in a travel clinic prior to departure to ensure they receive all necessary vaccinations and prophylaxis as well as instruction on the use of insect repellant and bed nets to avoid vector-borne diseases (Sarfaty and Arnold 2005). Other health precautions should also be discussed including general food preparation (such as avoidance of undercooked or raw meat, uncooked vegetables and fruit that cannot be peeled) as well as good hygienic practice (such as proper hand washing technique and use of hand sanitizer). Awareness must be raised about the risks associated with untreated tap and/or well water for items such as ice and fruit juice or for purposes of brushing teeth.

Students and residents should also meet with occupational health to discuss potential hazards, such as exposure to serious infections like tuberculosis, HIV, hepatitis B and C (Gardner et al. 2011). Provision of a basic medical kit and HIV post exposure prophylaxis (PEP) would also be prudent.

Student and residents should also be educated about the safety profile of the country to be visited. This should include general road traffic safety, particularly given that traffic accidents are one of the highest causes of mortality and morbidity worldwide with the risk for travelers equaling that of local populations (Sarfaty and Arnold 2005). Many countries often lack the infrastructure, resources, laws, and regulations necessary to ensure safe travel. As a result, roads may be in poor condition without lighting, while public transportation, including taxis and buses, may not be properly maintained. Furthermore, seat belts and helmets are often unavailable. These countries also have a greater number of people living in poverty, thus travelers who find themselves suddenly on unfamiliar terrain may be at increased risk for crime. While political instability and turmoil often can be anticipated, plans for regrouping and possible evacuation should be thoroughly discussed. While one can take measures to decrease the risk of such events, unanticipated injury, harm or illness may still occur. Therefore, programs should encourage both travel and evacuation insurance for all students.

It is imperative that all students have an understanding of the general political, historical, social, and cultural factors that shape the lives of people to be encountered both within and beyond the clinical setting (Crump and Sugarman 2010; Peluso et al. 2012; Taylor 1994). Programs should provide students and residents with a brief seminar on the most pertinent topics. Furthermore, it should be the goal of all participants to acquire at least basic language skills in order to integrate more fully as a healthcare provider and to gain a deeper understanding of cultural norms and practices (Crump and Sugarman 2010; Peluso et al. 2012; Taylor 1994). Effective language learning materials and tools should be identified so that all participants may begin efforts to learn the language in advance of their departure. Additionally, the host institution may arrange interpreter services for participants during their clinical hours.

Orientation Packet

Participants should be provided with an orientation packet containing a brief guide to the country including a summary of its history, government, geography and culture, a list of useful phrases in the local languages, and a reference of relevant books, music, film, and resources. The orientation packet should also include the following specifics regarding the international site: travel information (visas and passports, buses, trains, taxis, car rentals); health information (immunizations and medications); financial matters (exchange rates, general costs of living, access to banks and ATMs); accommodations and utilities (water, electricity, kitchenware and appliances); dining and self-catering options (markets, restaurants, grocery stores); communications (mobile phones and internet); safety concerns (how to avoid becoming a target, role of police enforcement in country, emergency contact numbers); tourism.

In-Country Preparation of US Trainees

Welcome Orientation

Arrangements should be made for participants to be met by a member of the global health office at the airport in order to display their support of the participants. A welcome orientation should be conducted for all students and residents. This enables the participants to have a smoother assimilation as they get their bearings in a new environment. This should include a review of pertinent information covered within the orientation packet, a discussion revolving around goals and expectations, a tour of the facility and accommodations, a meet and greet with key members of the global health office and medical community. Participants should also be linked as soon after arrival as possible with an individual who will be the contact person in the event of any issues or concerns that arise (Crump and Sugarman 2010).

Define Responsibilities and Expectations of Participants

A written contract with clear delineation of roles and expectations should be given to participants and serves multiple purposes (Crump and Sugarman 2010). It informs participants of what the program expects of them and what they can expect in return. Towards this end, the contract should include participant responsibilities while in the workplace: performing history and physical exams, rounding and pre-rounding, attendance and participation in conferences, codes of conduct, professionalism and dress code, work hours and schedules.

The terms of the contract should also set forth precautions against medical tourism, which can result in an experience with no direct bearing on participant professional development and with minimal-to-no benefit to the host site (Parsi and List 2008).

Furthermore, the contract should serve to protect vulnerable populations, be it patients who come under the participants' care or participants who are in a position to deliver that care. Students and residents interested in global health are guided by a strong sense of duty to serve in whatever capacity they can, though they may be unaware of their limitations (Crump and Sugarman 2010). Often in international settings, students and residents are given more patient responsibilities with less supervision potentially leading to adverse outcomes for both patient and provider (Axt et al. 2013). It is important to educate participants about their exact role in patient care and to ensure that standards of care are maintained, particularly given that no clear ethical guidelines exist for global health experiences for the protection of patients (Shah and Wu 2008). For example, given that students are not experienced in performing any procedures, they should not do so in any country without proper supervision.

Other expectations to note include acknowledgment and acceptance of specific health measures, such as adherence to anti-malarial prophylaxis, abiding to safety measures, such as registration with embassies, and communicating with the global health office for all in-country travel.

Curriculum at International Sites

Global health rotations are generally scheduled in 4–6 week blocks. Selected residents and students should undergo a comprehensive curriculum including direct patient care in the clinics and on the wards along with didactic sessions coupled with language and cultural classes.

Clinical Work

The opportunity should be available for participants to work in inpatient and outpatient settings as well as general and specialty services, though specific rotations will depend upon the arrangements made with the host institution. Programs often devise a single generic scheduling template for all participants made up of required blocks as well as electives to be tailored to individualized interests. Some medical specialties, such as palliative care or geriatrics, may enable participants to make home visits with a medical team and provide a rich context within which to frame patients and their illnesses.

Didactic Sessions

Students and residents will benefit from didactic sessions prepared and delivered by local experts with knowledge in important topics such as basic epidemiologic principles, medical education, healthcare delivery and insurance structure, and tropical medicine. A weekly session in parasitology lab could also be created for students and residents to become better versed in laboratory diagnosis of tropical diseases.

Cultural, Sociopolitical, and Language Curriculum

Over the duration of the rotation, participants should be offered a curriculum on the historical, cultural, and sociopolitical aspects of the country (Crump and Sugarman 2010). Faculty members from the host institution with expertise in these areas should be identified to help create the curriculum and to lead the discussion. In addition, an experienced language instructor should provide language classes multiple times a week. In the event that host families are available, participants would gain even greater language and cultural immersion.

Field Trips

Group excursions to visit important sites and attractions serves the role of supplementing the historical, cultural, and sociopolitical curriculum and rounding out participants' experience of the country and its people. Ideally, these organized trips can be scheduled during weekends during which no clinical duties are taking place and be led by members of the community who are familiar with the sites to be visited.

Research

Academic collaborations with strong components of clinical work and education are well poised to conduct research with direct bearing on the lives of patients. Institutions should not miss the opportunity to interface between these three elements and to discover innovative ways to deliver better care to patients.

Participants wishing to undertake a research project must begin planning months in advance of their trip. A research advisor should be identified to help the participant through all steps of the process. These may include a thorough literature review, generation of a feasible research question, submission of all relevant paperwork for both home and host institution ethics and/or Institutional Review Board (IRB) committees, outlining an expense report in the event that travel and research funds are available, procuring any necessary equipment, and most importantly, identifying a research mentor at the host institution. Alternatively, participants may also join up with an ongoing research project at the host institution on which to dedicate one's efforts given the typically short span of time in-country. Participants should submit a written report of some kind describing the work achieved, whether in the form of a scientific article or general report.

Of note, international research should be conducted after careful deliberation of the ethics involved to avoid exploitation of the vulnerable, to minimize risk to participants, and to provide benefit to the local population (Iserson et al. 2012). Lapses in research ethics may occur due to absence or inexperience by oversight committees in resource-limited settings or lack of insight into the values and needs of local communities by home institutions. As a result, researchers must remain vigilant and cognizant of these challenges whenever performing research abroad.

Accommodations

There are many options when it comes to accommodations. Participants may live on-campus, off-campus, alone, with other program participants or with a host family. There are many advantages of living with members of the local community, most importantly greater integration into the cultural, social and language components of the international experience. Students and residents living with members of the community can more effectively acquire both the linguistic skills as well as the cultural competence in order to have a more productive stay. With the caveat that steps are taken to select a safe neighborhood, living with members of the community generally offers greater security given that one is identified as being a part of the community and thus is absorbed into that network. The opportunity for communal dining experiences offers both a practical advantage as well as another avenue to immerse oneself in the local culture.

Identifying members specifically from the medical and academic community who can provide accommodations offers an additional benefit that bears mentioning. Not only would participants be privy to the kind of cultural and language immersion as previously discussed, but they would be able to engage with their host in a meaningful mentor-mentee relationship and feel anchored to a support system that can help alleviate emotional challenges related to their experiences.

Disadvantages of living with a host family often stem from intrinsic differences between the cultures of the participants and that of the community. Many cultures do not endorse the concept of the individual as much as they do that of the community. This cultural attribute may manifest itself in a lack of privacy and boundaries, which often proves difficult for those coming from a more individualistic culture. Specifically, one may be sharing a bedroom and/or bathroom with members of the host family. As a result, participants may not be afforded much time to themselves as most activities, including meals and recreation, are enjoyed collectively.

Conversely, living with other participants or alone offers greater independence. Students and residents are able to make their own schedules and have more flexibility with their day-to-day routine. They are also afforded more privacy.

The main disadvantage of living with other participants or alone is the social and cultural isolation given that it is more difficult to integrate with the local community. Participants will have greater difficulty learning a new language when placed in situations where they can readily converse in English as well as greater difficulty understanding unwritten local cultural and social norms. It is possible, however, for students to limit the extent of this isolation by putting more effort into seeking out the company of community members. In terms of safety, living on-campus usually has the benefit of reliable institutional security services, but in some countries it can also be the setting of unpredictable political turmoil and social unrest.

Evaluation and Quality Improvement

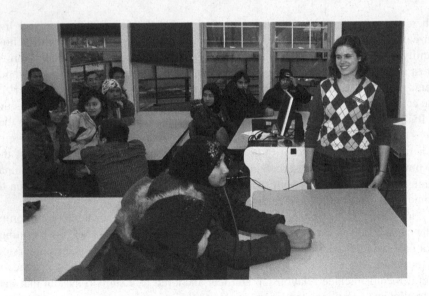

Weekly Feedback Sessions and Counseling

Participants will invariably have a range of experience in an international setting and subsequently may require different levels and types of support for the duration of their trip. It is essential to provide a setting in which they can readily and easily converse about their experiences. Also, particularly in the beginning stages of a collaboration, there undoubtedly will be programmatic kinks to work out. For these reasons, well-conducted weekly feedback and counseling sessions are paramount to the success of any partnership (Crump and Sugarman 2010; Peluso et al. 2012). Efforts should be made to identify an individual who can most effectively conduct these sessions. Desirable attributes include warmth and compassion, good communication skills, proficiency in English, a leader in the community with ample knowledge of the roles and responsibilities played by participants and experience working with people from different cultural backgrounds. Often it is useful to provide training on the concept of feedback given that this may not be a shared norm between cultures.

These weekly sessions serve multiple purposes. First, they provide feedback about the logistical components of the rotation, e.g., difficulties with accommodations, travel to and from housing to the hospital. Second, they provide feedback about work-related activities, e.g., whether there is ample autonomy in patient care, supervision, and teaching. Third, these sessions gauge participants' overall integration and level of contentment. The most effective way to begin these conversations is with open-ended questions such as, "How are things going overall?" Often there are events and goings-on of great influence to participants that may not be readily apparent and may be most easily elicited in this manner. On the other hand, there may be public events, such as planned political demonstrations or religious holidays, which can be more directly addressed. In the event that there is concern that one or more of the participants is feeling overwhelmed and is in need of more time to discuss specific events and situations, time can be allotted either singly or in groups, as appropriate.

Mid-rotation and End-of-Rotation Evaluations

The purpose of mid-rotation and end-of-rotation evaluation is twofold: (1) to provide feedback to participants about what they are doing well and what requires further improvement; (2) to receive feedback from participants about what specifics of the program are working well and what requires improvement. A formal feedback and evaluation tool should be designed to provide a standardized framework. Programs should identify one member of the host institution who can provide mid-rotation and end-of-rotation feedback to participants. Generally, the program director is in a good position to take on this role given that they will have received training in the United States, including the methods of delivering appropriate and timely feedback. It is important that this individual not be directly supervising participants, but rather well informed of participants' clinical performances as well as contributions in other areas, including didactics, language, and cultural sessions.

Debriefing

It is important to offer post-rotation debriefing to the group in order to discuss the experience in its entirety and identify any specific aspects of the rotation that participants wish to discuss (Crump and Sugarman 2010).

Program Evaluation and Feedback

Participants can offer great insight into the ways in which specific aspects of the program are meeting or falling short of general objectives as well as into their levels of satisfaction. One effective way of acquiring this information in a quantitative manner is through participants' involvement with program evaluation and feedback (Peluso et al. 2012). More qualitative information can be obtained by requesting participants to write a paper describing not only the work they accomplished, but also to reflect on the meaning of their experiences (Taylor 1994).

Continuous Quality Improvement

It should be a priority of the program to make frequent and honest assessments of all aspects of the collaboration to ensure that its mission is preserved and its goals and objectives met. A committee with members from both sites should be formed and tasked with the evaluation of the program on a regular basis. Steps should be taken to identify ways in which the program is meeting or failing to meet specific goals and objectives. Interventions must then be executed that would allow the program to remedy any shortcomings.

Measurement of specific outcomes can be achieved through use of biometrics. For example, in determining overall impact of a global health program on students and residents, one can conduct pre- and post-rotation evaluations on knowledge base, such as tropical medicine, as well as clinical skills, such as cultural competence and empathy.

While it is essential to quantify outcomes and determine the overall success of the program, it must be noted that some of the more profound impact generated from global health programs requires a different form of measurement. It takes patience to invest in the potential of individuals and to await the outcome of that investment. One must consider medical students and residents who are awakened to truths about the human condition, the systems impacting that condition, and the resolve they experience when they visualize the role they can play in bringing about needed change. One must consider young faculty members who develop prowess in the field of medicine and return to their homes and communities charged with new energy and novel ideas. The changes arising within each of these individuals become the catalyst to help so many others who are within the sphere of influence of these future leaders.

Challenges

Preservation of Dignity of Host Institution

The principle of paramount importance to abide by while constructing and delivering a global health program is to protect and preserve the dignity of the host institution (Crump and Sugarman 2010). This is about them, only then can it be about us. Towards this end, one must avoid situations of exploitation and prioritize efforts towards capacity building and sustainability (Iserson et al. 2012). Given the dynamic nature of healthcare delivery and cross-cultural exchanges, one must continually evaluate all dimensions of the program and make any necessary adjustments to ensure that local needs are being met and that all activities are of benefit to the host site. A focus on capacity building and sustainability not only takes into account the identification and optimization of available resources, but also aims to avoid drawing away of resources and personnel from where they are most needed.

Need for Cultural Grace

Unfortunately, there are some individuals who, despite appropriate fund of knowledge and clinical acumen, and likely with no intention, are capable of inflicting harm so severe to test even the strongest collaboration. Much of this harm is rooted in a sense of entitlement or a general lack of cultural grace in which inflexibility mars cultural understanding. These individuals, led by a brazen notion of infallibility, act without any attempt at understanding the tremendous consequences of their actions on their colleagues, patients, hosts and medical community, even citing patient advocacy as underlying their actions. Yet patient advocacy cannot exist in the vacuum of ethnocentricity and blossoms only with great care to a place and its people. What is at stake is the trust that at once binds the partners and upon which any hope of success pivots. Thus, it becomes crucial to the partnership that participants be selected with this attribute in mind. Efforts should be made to prepare and orient these individuals as much as possible to their new setting and open lines of communication should be put in place to address any matters of concern. If these efforts fail, one must stand firm on immediate dismissal of the individual who brings disgrace to the program.

Funding

For the academic and medical institutions in the United States, procurement of sufficient support, both financial and otherwise, remains an obstacle (Francis et al. 2012). The creation and growth of a global health program requires a great deal of institutional investment, both in terms of time and resources. Given the pronounced influence of global health programs on the motivations of medical students and residents and the particular role to be played by medical universities in training the next generation of global health leaders, the onus of providing the financial backing for these programs primarily falls on the American medical institution itself. This financial investment extends beyond a mere fiscal decision to a sense of stewardship on the part of the medical institution towards the enterprise of global health.

Once the institution has taken on global health programming, steps should be taken towards sustainability of the program (Castillo et al. 2012; Campagna et al. 2013). Efforts of acquiring further funding can be made through various avenues such as securement of private donations, governmental grants, and providing a service worthy of tuition. For example, the need for a global health program at other medical education institutions that lack both the experience and sufficient funding to establish their own program makes them amenable to paying a tuition fee to collaborate with an institution with a successful program. Programs can also establish visitor medical education (VME) programs for highly or moderately developed countries to provide an additional source of funding. A well-devised and well-publicized VME program may be crucial in the sustainability of a global health program, and once set in motion, will lend a more robust international community to the academic campus.

Emotional Wellbeing

Culture shock is a phenomenon that occurs frequently and can vary from drastic to more commonplace. It also can impact various aspects of life and living. It is a particularly difficult process with which to grapple when placed in the context of resource-limited settings. With support and an outlet to speak candidly about the gamut of feelings that culture shock elicits, many participants are able to move towards a meaningful and productive experience (Sarfaty and Arnold 2005).

The main challenge posed by culture shock lies at its extreme, where travelers lose the ability to ground their experiences and become subjected to emotional exhaustion (Sarfaty and Arnold 2005). No matter how much preparation or prior experience participants may have, they will inevitably shoulder a daily grind, both minute and grand, pertaining to both the culture of medicine and life circumstances. These unremitting moments, which find participants struggling to make sense of unembellished and stark renderings of tragedy, are taxing at a minimum. At their most damaging, these moments can be crippling and may lead participants to a sense of futility and loss of hope. This threat must be engaged seriously and competently by members of global health programs by careful consideration of the methods employed to reduce the burden of emotional exhaustion in the participants. For this reason, it must be emphasized that supervision of participants necessarily falls to members of the medical community who will take a vested interest in the overall wellbeing of participants and who understand the weight of their role in mentorship and guidance. It is also possible to monitor participants' periods of adjustment through the use of daily journaling and weekly reflections. By spending an hour per day recording their thoughts, participants can more readily fall into a habit of self-reflection. These entries are to remain personal, though the weekly reflections may be submitted and used to gauge how students are coping with their experiences. Interestingly, participants' written thoughts take on a transparency that helps program administrations identify who may require early intervention in the form of counseling to prevent emotional exhaustion.

Upon their return to the United States, travelers may undergo a similar process of reverse culture shock or "reentry shock" (Sarfaty and Arnold 2005). Having witnessed crippling poverty and unstifled acts of injustice, participants undergo a difficult transition period as they attempt to come to terms with the stark contrast between the conditions of peoples' lives and fortunes in these two different settings. When seeking friends and family with whom to discuss these issues, they are often met with ambivalence or even disinterest. Given that many travelers deem reverse culture shock as the more challenging period of transition, participants should be prepared as much as possible with ample support provided at their home institutions.

Conclusion and Future Direction

Enthusiasm around global health is burgeoning across medical institutions. In the hands of medical students, residents and faculty members, this enthusiasm sends forth new growth in every direction from border medicine near Mexico to teaching the first class of medical students in Africa's newest nation, South Sudan. More students are entering the field of medicine versed in the language of global health and equipped to take on roles with social and humanistic dimensions. They look to institutional administrators to not only provide them with avenues to engage this interest, but to exemplify the goals and vision of the global health movement. In the face of this momentous expectation, program leadership has an opportunity to guide the next generation of citizens of the world: individuals who will become leaders in global health, creators of scientific knowledge, and instruments of change in the dispelling of disparities.

Towards this goal, academic institutions must mount a thoughtful, well-structured global health program both within and beyond their campuses with like-minded partners. These partnerships, when led by multidisciplinary and longitudinal efforts aimed at sustainability and mutual benefit, will reach their promise and cultivate the concept of being "more for them than for us."

As the landscape of global health changes so does the relationship of academic centers with that landscape. The rigorous use of biometrics and other methods in the continuous evaluation of interventions and their outcomes aims to ascribe transparency to collaborative endeavors and to ensure flexibility in more effectively addressing program goals within this shifting landscape. A measured and exacting approach to the selection of program participants purports to identify those with cultural grace who will be true ambassadors of global health rather than those still entrenched in principles of colonialism. Providing a sound infrastructure built on appropriate supervision and attention to emotional health will ensure the safety of participants and the quality of the overall experience.

As programs expand and strengthen their foundation, they must focus on providing opportunities for students and residents to acquire and hone qualities of leadership. Adding an outreach component to a global health program is one such avenue. During outreach work, participants begin from the grassroots level, visiting people's homes and communities, listening and learning, finding a place amongst the people, and building relationships. From this vantage point, they are able to assess community health needs, find solutions with real likelihood of success, implement interventions aimed at bolstering the health of the community, and preventing unacceptable health outcomes. This model of outreach envisions not just the health of individuals but the health of a community as a living organism. The mobilization of a community towards a thriving state demands a wide array of skills. One must possess knowledge of medicine and public health, awareness of the socio-cultural and political underpinnings of health in specific communities, language and communication abilities, dexterity with tools of social media, and the ability to identify and engage with community leaders and group organizers. One also requires the imagination and adeptness to conceive of the potential in collaboration with academic centers, governmental and non-governmental organizations in order to reach establish goals.

The importance of investing in this cohort of leaders in global health is particularly evident when considering human populations pushed to the farthest recesses of inequality. The intolerable state of health in these communities often is a result of a confluence of historical, political, and scientific factors that demands greater efforts of understanding as well as greater commitment to action. It is at this junction, wherein the most neglected reside, that one finds not only the greatest challenges of medicine but also the greatest optimism—in the potential of the next leaders in global health and in the promise of real change.

References

Association of American Medical Colleges (2012) 2012 Medical School Graduation Questionnaire All Schools Summary Report. Association of American Medical Colleges, Washington, DC. https://www.aamc.org/download/300448/data. Accessed July 2012

Axt J, Nthuma PM, Mwanzia K, Hansen E, Tarpley MJ, Krishnaswami S, Nwomeh BC, Holterman A, Hadler EP, Simione D, Orloff S, Tarpley JL, Merchant NB (2013) Commentary: the role of global surgery electives during residency training: relevance, realities, and regulations. Surgery 153:327–332

Balandin S, Lincoln M, Sen R, Wilkins DP, Trembath D (2007) Twelve tips for effective international clinical placements. Med Teach 29:872–877

Beaglehole R, Bonita R (2010) Editorial: what is global health? Glob Health Action 3:5142. doi:10.3402/gha.v3i0.5142 3: 5142

Campagna AM, Clair NE, Gladding SP, Wagner SM, John CC (2013) Essential factors for the development of a residency global health track. Clin Pediatr 52(9):862–871

Castillo J, Castillo H, Ayoub-Rodriguez L, Jennings JE, Jones K, Oliver S, Schubert CJ, Dewitt T (2012) The resident decision-making process in global health education. Clin Pediatr 51:462

Crump JA, Sugarman J (2010) Working Group on Ethics Guidelines for Global Health Training (WEIGHT). Ethics and best practice guidelines for training experiences in global health. Am J Trop Med Hyg 83(6):1178–1182

Drain PK, Primack A, Hunt DD, Fawzi WW, Holmes KK, Gardner P (2007) Global health in medical education: a call for more training and opportunities. Acad Med Mar 82(3):226–230

Fineberg HV, Hunter DJ (2013) Editorial: a global view of health. N Engl J Med 368:78–79

Francis ER, Goodsmith N, Michelow M, Kulkarni A, McKenney AS, Kishore SP, Bertelsen N, Fein O, Salsari S, Lemery J, Fitzgerald D, Johnson W, Finkel ML (2012) The global health curriculum of Weill Cornell Medical College: how one school developed a global health program. Acad Med 87(9):1296–1302

Frenk J, Chen L, Bhutta ZA, Cohen J, Crisp N, Evans T, Fineberg H, Garcia P, Ke Y, Kelley P, Kistnasamy B, Meleis A, Naylor D, Pablos-Mendez A, Reddy S, Scrimshaw S, Sepulveda J, Serwadda D, Zurayk H (2010) Health professionals for a new century: transforming education to strengthen health systems in an interdependent world. Lancet 376(9756):1923–1958

Gardner A, Cohen T, Carter EJ (2011) Tuberculosis among participants in an academic global health medical exchange program. J Gen Intern Med 26(8):841–845

Garfunkel LC, Howard CR (2011) Expand education in global health: it is time. Acad Pediatr 11:260–262

Goldner BW, Bollinger RC (2012) Global health education for medical students: new learning opportunities and strategies. Med Teach 23:e58–e63

Iserson KV, Biros MH, Holiman CJ (2012) Challenges in international medicine: ethical dilemmas, unanticipated consequences, and accepting limitations. Acad Emerg Med 19:683–692

Kickbusch I (2006) The need for a European strategy on global health. Scand J Pub Health 34:561–565

Koplan JP, Bond TC, Merson MH, Reddy KS, Rodriguez MH, Sewankambo NK et al (2009) Towards a common definition of global health. Lancet 373:1993–1995

Mao JJ, Wax J, Barg FK, Margo K, Walrath D (2007) A gain in cultural competence through an international acupuncture elective. Fam Med 39(1):16–18

Nakanjako D, Byakika-Kibwika P, Kintu K, Aizire J, Nakwagala F, Luzige S, Namisi C, Mayanja-Kizza H, Kamya MR (2011) Mentorship needs at academic institutions in resource-limited settings: a survey at Makerere University College of Health Sciences. Med Educ 11:53

Nelson BD, Saltzman A, Lee PT (2012) Bridging the global health training gap: design and evaluation of a new clinical global health course at Harvard Medical School. Med Teach 34:45–51

Parsi K, List J (2008) Preparing medical students for the world: service learning and global health justice. Medscape J Med 10(11):268. Epub 2008 Nov 25

Peluso MJ, Encandela J, Hafler JP, Margolis CZ (2012) Guiding principles for the development of global health education curricular in undergraduate medical education. Med Teach 23:653–658

Peluso MJ, Forrestel AK, Hafler JP, Rohrbaugh RM (2013) Structured global health programs in U.S. medical schools: a web-based review of certificates, tracks, and concentrations. Acad Med 88(1):124–130

Rabin TL, Schwartz J (2012) The global health chief resident: modifying an established role, strengthening a collaboration. Med Educ 46(11):1128–1129

Ramsey AH, Haq C, Gjerde CL, Rothenberg D (2004) Career influence of an international health experience during medical school. Fam Med 36(6):412–416

Sarfaty S, Arnold LK (2005) Preparing for international medical service. Emerg Med Clin North Am 23(1):149–175

Shah S, Wu T (2008) The medical student global health experience: professionalism and ethical implications. J Med Ethics 34(5):375–378

Smith JK, Weaver DB (2006) Capturing medical students' idealism. Ann Fam Med 4(Suppl 1): S32–S37; discussion S58–60

Taylor CE (1994) International experience and idealism in medical education. Acad Med 69(8):631–634

Wilson JW, Merry SP, Franz WB (2012) Rules of engagement: the principles of underserved global health volunteerism. Am J Med 125:613–617

Chapter 15
Assessing Student Performance

Brian Mavis

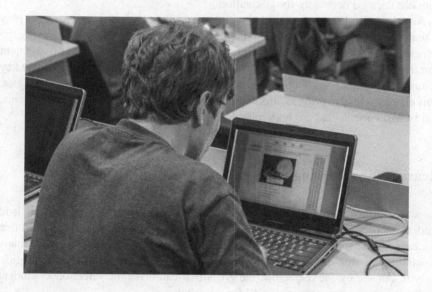

Abstract Assessment bridges the gap between teaching and learning. Perhaps second only to teaching, assessing student performance is a fundamental role in the life of a teacher. Assessment is important because it provides students with feedback about their performance; this information reinforces their areas of strength and highlights areas of weakness. Using this feedback, students can direct their study strategies and seek additional resources to improve their performance.

B. Mavis, Ph.D. (✉)
OMERAD (Office of Medical Education Research and Development),
Michigan State University College of Human Medicine,
965 Fee Road, Room A202, East Lansing, MI 48824, USA
e-mail: mavis@msu.edu

K.N. Huggett and W.B. Jeffries (eds.), *An Introduction to Medical Teaching*,
DOI 10.1007/978-94-017-9066-6_15, © Springer Science+Business Media Dordrecht 2014

Introduction

Assessment bridges the gap between teaching and learning. Perhaps second only to teaching, assessing student performance is a fundamental role in the life of a teacher. Assessment is important because it provides students with feedback about their performance; this information reinforces their areas of strength and highlights areas of weakness. Using this feedback, students can direct their study strategies and seek additional resources to improve their performance.

From the perspective of the teacher, another equally important function of student assessment is providing evidence necessary for decisions about student progress. The various student assessments within a class define the types and levels of achievement expected of students. As part of a course of study, student assessments describe a developmental process of increasing competency across a range of domains deemed necessary for graduation.

Any thoughtful teacher realizes the important role that student assessments play in their lives as teachers as well as in the lives of their students. Less obvious are the principles of educational measurement underlying sound student assessment practices. The purpose of this chapter is to provide an overview of some of the key features to consider when choosing among various student assessment strategies. This chapter will also provide information on how to create fair student assessments, that is, assessments that are both reliable and valid.

Reasons for Assessing Student Performance

As stated above, the assessment of student performance provides feedback to students about what they have or have not learned, and provides information that teachers can use in student progress decisions. However, these are only two of many possible goals that can influence your selection of student assessment strategies. As you can see by the list below, the goals that can drive the selection of student performance measures are many and far reaching:

- Providing feedback to students about their mastery of course content
- Grading or ranking students for progress and promotion decisions
- Offering encouragement and support to students (or teachers)
- Measuring changes in knowledge, skills or attitudes over time
- Diagnosing weaknesses in student performance
- Establishing performance expectations for students
- Identifying areas for improving instruction
- Documenting instructional outcomes for faculty promotion
- Evaluating the extent that educational objectives are realized
- Encouraging the development of a new curriculum
- Demonstrating quality standards for the public, institution or profession
- Articulating the values and priorities of the educational institution
- Informing the allocation of educational resources

Clearly, many of these goals are related directly to the interaction between teacher and student. Nonetheless, this same information can be used by other stakeholders in the educational process for a variety of other important decisions (Shumway and Harden 2003). From a practical perspective, it is unlikely that any single assessment strategy can provide information to support more than a few of these goals. The likelihood for misinterpretation or inaccuracy increases when student assessment data are used for purposes other than those originally intended. The sheer breadth of the list of goals above also demonstrates the importance of considering the use of multiple strategies to assess student learning.

In the curriculum development cycle presented in Chap. 12, student assessment follows instruction and is the impetus for reflection, evaluation and curricular improvement. While this cycle might reflect how many teachers approach teaching, from the student perspective, it is the assessment phase of the curriculum that drives learning. This is most often manifest when students ask, "do we have to know this for the test?" For many students their motivation is survival, and in an educational setting, one key element of survival is passing the test, whatever form student assessments might take. This is particularly true when results from assessments will be used for decisions about student progress or other high-stakes outcomes.

Learning the Language of Assessment: A Few Definitions

Before getting much deeper into a discussion of student assessment, it is important that we clarify a few definitions of key terms and their meaning in this context.

Assessment Versus Evaluation

Both assessment and evaluation refer to processes of gathering information for the purposes of decision-making. In medical education, assessment most often refers to the measurement of individual student performance, while evaluation refers to the measurement of outcomes for courses, educational programs or institutions. Practically speaking, students are assessed while educational programs are evaluated. However, it is often the case that aggregated student assessments serve as an important information source when evaluating educational programs.

Formative Versus Summative Assessment

Formative assessments are used to give students feedback about their learning. Practice test questions or problem sets, in-class peer-graded assignments and reviews of video recorded simulated patient encounters are examples of frequently used formative assessment strategies. Formative assessments are most valuable when they are separated from summative assessments, so that they are perceived to be low threat performance experiences. For conscientious students, this represents an opportunity to document both strengths and weaknesses. However, some students might dismiss formative assessments for their lack of consequences, and not put their best effort forward to use these experiences to maximal advantage.

Summative assessments are used to gather information to judge student achievement and to make student progress decisions (Miller et al., 1998). These assessments are very familiar to students and teachers, and for students often provoke anxiety. A substantial component of this anxiety comes from the student progress decisions predicated on performance. However, to the extent that uncertainty about the summative assessment strategy itself is a source of anxiety, teachers can take steps to reduce student anxiety. This includes providing information about the types of assessments to be used, their timing within a course, how they are scored and how each contributes to the final grade or progress decision. Students often become anxious in an unfamiliar assessment situation, such as a standardized patient encounter or new computer-based testing software. Sample interactions, in-class demonstrations or opportunities for non-graded practice can help students anticipate what to expect under these circumstances, which might help reduce their anxiety.

Ideally, learning situations provide students with multiple opportunities for both formative and summative feedback (Amin et al., 2006). Formative feedback helps students *improve* their learning while summative feedback allows them to *prove* their learning. In practice, educators tend to focus on summative assessment, sometimes with little or no attention paid to providing opportunities for formative assessment. The obvious reason for this imbalance is the need to document learning for progress decisions, which is often coupled with limited instructor time and resources available for developing formative assessments. It is also true that many instructors do not appreciate the importance of practice in the context of formative assessment as a powerful tool to promote learning.

Competence

It is increasingly common in medical education for discussions of student assessment to lead to discussions of competence. One current definition of competence provided by Epstein and Hundert (2002) gives us a sense of the tip of the iceberg implied by these discussions. They wrote that "*professional competence is the habitual and judicious use of communication, knowledge, technical skills, clinical reasoning, emotions, values and reflection in daily practice for the benefit of the individual and community being served.*" From the practical perspective of an educator, competence requires us to set expectations of satisfactory performance appropriate for the students' progress within the curriculum.

A number of developmental models useful to learner assessment have been described. One important hierarchical model of competence was articulated by George Miller (1990), who described a developmental approach that is helpful when thinking about appropriate forms of learner assessment. For novice learners, competence is determined by what students *know*, i.e., their mastery of factual knowledge. At the next level, competence is defined by an assessment requiring students to demonstrate what they *know how* to do, such as how to use and apply knowledge to solve new problems, or demonstrate the clinical skills necessary to gather clinical data. Assessments at the next level, *showing how,* require students to actually demonstrate their ability to acquire, interpret and translate knowledge. At the highest level of competence, students would demonstrate competence by *doing*, which would be assessments of how they perform in an encounter with a patient in a real world setting.

Another developmental approach useful for learner assessment and feedback is the RIME model, originally developed for use in clinical settings (Sepdham et al., 2007). RIME is the acronym for the four levels of performance outlined by the model: reporter, interpreter, manager and educator. Each level describes increasing degrees of sophistication of a student's ability to collect and synthesize clinical data. Learners progress from being able to *report* data with an understanding of the nature of the patient's problems, to being able to *interpret* the data and understand possible causes of the patient's problem. At the *manager* level, students demonstrate an understanding of how to treat the problem, while *educators* can generalize their learning to more complicated problems and contribute to the continued learning of the health care team. Some versions of this model include *observer* as the initial stage prior to *reporter* when the student has not yet developed data gathering skills.

Key Features of Student Assessment Methods

There are a number of factors to consider when choosing a method of student assessment. Attention to these factors at the planning stage will go a long way to helping you create a high quality student assessment. Five factors to consider are:

1. Reliability
2. Validity
3. Feasibility
4. Acceptability
5. Educational Impact

Reliability and validity are characteristics that generally refer to the process used to develop an assessment. Feasibility, acceptability and educational impact more often reflect contextual features of the assessment, which are related to when and how an assessment method is implemented (Mehrens and Lehmann 1991).

Reliability

When talking about an assessment method in terms of reliability, we are referring to the consistency or repeatability of measurement. In practice a reliable assessment should yield the same result when given to the same student at two different times or by two different examiners. One of the advantages of tests comprised of multiple-choice questions is that they are highly reliable: the results of the test are unlikely to be influenced by when the test is administered, when the test is scored or by who does the scoring. Hence the term "objective" is often used when referring to these kinds of assessments. On the other hand, reliability is an important concern when grading essay questions, rating clinical skills or scoring other assessments requiring judgment or interpretation. In these situations, clear scoring criteria are needed to attain a high level of reliability, regardless of whether one or multiple people will be involved in grading the responses. Writing clear questions and instructions is another important strategy for improving the reliability of an assessment by reducing the likelihood that test questions or assessment tasks are ambiguous to the reader and open to interpretation. Writing clear test questions also increases the likelihood that the assessment is testing desired knowledge, skills or attitudes rather than reading proficiency or verbal reasoning skills.

Internal consistency is another form of reliability that is frequently used to describe assessments based on multiple-choice questions. This term refers to the coherence of the test items, or the extent to which the test questions are interrelated. The primary difference between this and other estimates of reliability is that calculations of internal consistency involve only one administration of the test. For example, a set of multiple choice questions focused on assessing students' knowledge of childhood immunizations should have high internal consistency. When questions testing other knowledge or abilities are added, the internal consistency is lowered. Internal consistency estimates are frequently provided as part of the output for machine-scored multiple choice tests. The concept of internal consistency can be applied to other methods of assessment; this is best done in consultation with a measurement specialist.

Validity

Validity is the extent to which an assessment measures what it is intended to measure. Validity is related to reliability, insofar as a test that has low reliability will have limited validity. A test with low reliability is subject to biases in interpretation and scoring, and when these biases are unrelated to specific content or student perfor-mance, the validity of the assessment is diminished (Cook and Beckman 2006).

The validity of any assessment depends on the context in which it is implemented. An assessment validated in a specific context or with a specific learner group may be

Clinical Competency	Case 1	Case 2	Case 3	Case 4	Case 5	Case 6
Communication skills	x	x	x	x		x
History-taking		x	x	x		x
Physical examination		x	x	x		x
Data interpretation			x	x	x	
Assessment/Diagnosis			x	x	x	x
Patient education	x					
Written record	x		x	x	x	x

Fig. 15.1 Sample blueprint for a clinical competence examination

less valid when used in very different settings or other learner groups. The important message is that validity is context-specific and inferences based on data derived from one setting may be more or less valid than when the assessment is used in a different setting.

Among the many types of validity discussed in education and social science research, content validity is the approach most commonly used to assure quality in student assessment. Essentially, an assessment is valid when it samples representatively from the course content. A common method for assuring that the assessment content is representative of the course content is to develop a table of specifications, often referred to as a test blueprint. The blueprint organizes course content by course objectives, such as students' ability to recall factual information, understand concepts or apply knowledge to new problems. Another approach to organizing content could be based on patient cases (well child visit, asthma, developmental delay, etc.), or by disciplines (pathology, physiology, pharmacology, nutrition, etc.). In reality, any organizing structure that reflects the logic of the course content can be used as the basis of the blueprint (Fig. 15.1).

Ideally, the course content was initially designed around a blueprint based on the course objectives. In this way, the organization of the course informs the organization of the assessment content, creating a valid assessment (Anderson and Krathwohl 2001). In situations where there are no preexisting course objectives, it might be necessary to derive them from the content and reverse engineer a blueprint prior to creating the assessment.

Content based on a blueprint approach works well for assessments that focus on recall and application of knowledge. This approach also can be extended to assessments of clinical skills. The specific steps used to teach communication, history-taking and physical exam skills define the content, and a rating form can be developed to judge student performance of these skills. Another approach frequently used for the assessment of skills is expert judgment. A number of faculty members with expertise in the content area can be polled to determine what they would identify as the important content and this consensus is the basis for sampling content to assess student performance.

In general, sampling assessment content from the same blueprint that was used to define instructional content can enhance the validity of an assessment. Using multiple methods of assessment might be necessary when complex performance involving a combination of knowledge, attitudes and skills is the focus of assessment. Further, some assessment methods are more appropriate for some types of performance than others, so choosing appropriate methods can increase validity.

Feasibility

The feasibility of an assessment method is a judgment of the resources needed to implement it in light of the information to be gained. The development of a multiple choice test requires significant time in the development phase for question writing, but requires relatively little effort for administration or scoring. Conversely, a comprehensive assessment of clinical skills might require as many resources for scoring as for development and implementation, though the types of resources required might be different for each phase. Essentially, any assessment requires time for development, implementation and scoring. Additional resources might include examiners and/or simulated patients, as well as training time for each. Proctors, computers, biological samples, clinical case information, video recording facilities, curricular time and building space are among other possible resources that can facilitate or constrain an assessment.

Acceptability

Consider a teacher weighing the use of three assessment strategies: weekly tests, a more traditional mid-course and final exam, or a single cumulative examination at the end. Each approach has its merits as well as limitations, depending on the purpose of the assessment. The acceptability of an assessment is based on the responsiveness of faculty and students to the assessment. If the assessment requires too much time from faculty and staff or requires too many resources to implement, the long-term survival of the assessment is jeopardized. Similarly, an assessment approach might be aversive to students because of the timing, length, content or other features. When this occurs and students do not prepare as expected for the assessment or do not see it as valuable to their education, the validity of the assessment can be questioned.

Educational Impact

The educational impact of an assessment is the sum of many influences. The intent of the assessment relative to the course objectives is a consideration. The thoughtful use of both formative and summative assessments can positively affect student learning and subsequent student performance. Educational impact also reflects the appropriateness of the match between the content and the assessment method; a mismatch reduces the educational impact. Since content and assessment method are linked, the use of multiple assessment methods can enhance the impact. Relying on a single method tends to focus assessment on the content most amenable to the method. For example, the use of multiple choice questions favors the assessment of knowledge over skills. The method can also influence how students prepare for an assessment, such as the differences in preparation for a multiple choice exam versus an encounter with a standardized patient.

Choosing an Assessment Method

Consider this example. As part of the neuroscience curriculum, second-year medical students were asked to identify the location of a lesion based on a written case included as part of their final examination. The assessment was based on multiple choice questions. The correct response was chosen by 88 % of the class. The next day when the same written patient case was presented in a different format, within the context of a simulated patient encounter, only 35 % of the class got the answer correct. The conclusions about student performance based on each assessment would be very different. This example reflects the impact of assessment method in terms of both format and cognitive demands on the student.

When choosing an assessment method, there are several factors to consider. One of the first considerations is the type of performance to be assessed: is the assessment focusing on knowledge, skills or attitudes? Another factor that might influence the choice of assessment method is whether it is being used for formative or summative assessment. A related concern is the reliability and validity of the method. Some methods are more practical than others when considering the resources required to achieve reliable and valid results. Another consideration is whether more than one assessment approach should be used. When choosing an assessment method, it is important to remember that no single method "does it all." For this reason, a multiple-methods approach will probably provide a more accurate picture of student performance or achievement than relying on a single approach. As educators this idea makes intuitive sense; in practice we tend to stick to what is familiar.

Figure 15.2 summarizes the relative strengths of various assessment methods when measuring different types of performance. The chart provides guidance in choosing assessment methods, but is not intended to be absolute in matching methods and performance.

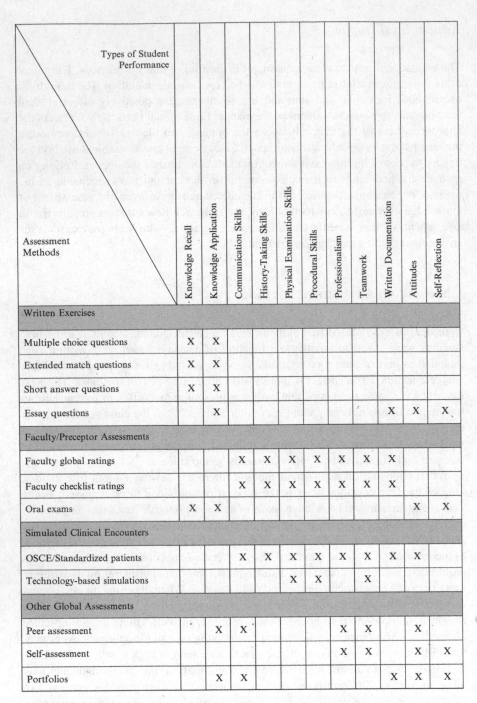

	Knowledge Recall	Knowledge Application	Communication Skills	History-Taking Skills	Physical Examination Skills	Procedural Skills	Professionalism	Teamwork	Written Documentation	Attitudes	Self-Reflection
Written Exercises											
Multiple choice questions	X	X									
Extended match questions	X	X									
Short answer questions	X	X									
Essay questions		X							X	X	X
Faculty/Preceptor Assessments											
Faculty global ratings			X	X	X	X	X	X	X		
Faculty checklist ratings			X	X	X	X	X	X	X		
Oral exams	X	X							X		X
Simulated Clinical Encounters											
OSCE/Standardized patients			X	X	X	X	X	X	X	X	
Technology-based simulations					X	X			X		
Other Global Assessments											
Peer assessment		X	X					X	X		X
Self-assessment								X	X		X	X
Portfolios		X	X						X	X	X

Fig. 15.2 Strengths of various assessment methods

Methods of Student Assessment

There is a wide range of methods available when developing your approach to student assessment, as shown in Fig. 15.2. These are the assessment methods most common to medical education and while not exhaustive, they represent a wide range of options available to faculty. The methods described in this section are organized into four broad categories: assessments based on written exercises, assessments derived from faculty ratings of performance, simulation-based assessments, and methods of global performance assessment. Each of the methods is described in terms of (a) strengths, (b) limitations, (c) reliability and validity and (d) construction tips.

Multiple Choice Questions (MCQ)

Assessments based on multiple choice questions (MCQ) are one of the most common approaches to measuring student performance. Typically, a multiple choice question consists of two parts: the question (stem) and the possible answers (response options). Most MCQs include four or five response options and the student is asked to choose the best response. The stem also can make reference to tables, graphs or other information sources that the student must use in order to determine the correct response.

Which of the following vitamins is involved in clotting factor synthesis?

(a) Vitamin A
(b) Vitamin B1
(c) Vitamin D
(d) Vitamin E
(e) Vitamin K

Strengths

- Multiple choice questions are familiar to most students, given their common usage throughout most levels of education.
- MCQs provide broad coverage of content: it is relatively easy to build an examination using MCQs that covers a wide range of course content.
- MCQs can be simply written to test for recall of factual knowledge, or can make reference to graphs, tables or illustrations to test cognitive skills. MCQs also can be posed within the context of a science problem or clinical case to test knowledge application and problem solving.
- Scoring of MCQs is highly reliable and objective.
- Scoring of MCQs can be automated, making scoring efficient and reducing the turnaround time for feedback to students. Automated scoring also facilitates the calculation of psychometric properties of each MCQ.

- MCQs are more flexible than True and False questions, which require absolute statements. MCQs are more flexible in terms of absolutes since the student is asked to choose the best answer from several possible options.

Limitations

- Good MCQs are challenging to write especially for applications beyond knowledge recall, such as knowledge application and problem solving. The time saved in scoring a MCQ examination is usually required up front in the preparation of the questions, requiring both time and careful consideration to avoid cueing students about the correct response option.
- MCQs frequently focus on recall of factual information and rely on students' recognition of the correct answer from among the options provided.
- Guessing can be a successful test-taking strategy for those questions where the student can rule out a number of the response options.
- MCQs are limited as a means of providing instructive feedback to students since usually the only information provided is the correct response option.
- The ease of use and economy of scoring associated with MCQs can lead to their overuse in situations when other types of assessment would be more appropriate.

Reliability and Validity

- Reliability tends not to be an issue for MCQs, which are the most frequently used objective test format. MCQ scoring is highly reliable in terms of consistency from one time to the next as might occur if the exams are scored over several sessions. Scoring is consistent between examiners; scoring of MCQs is not dependent on who is scoring the exams.
- Validity of an exam based on MCQs is enhanced through the use of a test blueprint, which assures that the distribution and coverage of examination content matches the instructional objectives and major content areas.

Construction Tips

- The response choices should be relatively brief, with the major content elements of the question included in the stem. The content can include graphs, images, clinical scenarios, research findings or other complex information that requires interpretation.
- Write each response option so that it matches the grammar of the stem.
- Equally distribute the position of the correct response across a series of questions. For example, the correct answer should not always be the third response option. A strategy to avoid such bias is to always order your response options alphabetically or numerically. Knowing this, the students cannot expect position bias.
- Do not use "all of the above" or "none of the above" as a response option.
- Avoid questions worded with negatives or double negatives.
- The correct and incorrect response options should be about the same length.
- Avoid the use of response options that are irrelevant or silly. This increases the likelihood of guessing the correct response.

- One MCQ can be viewed as a cluster of true/false questions, where one response choice is true and all of the others are false. When using true and false questions, the number of true and false questions should be roughly equal, and care should be used to construct questions of approximately the same length. A limitation of true and false questions is that for questions where the correct choice is false, you do not have assurance that the students in fact know the true answer. Another limitation of true and false questions is that they require statements that are absolutely true or absolutely false. These types of questions are best used for assessing factual recall.

Extended-Matching Questions

The extended-matching question format was developed to address some of the limitations of the MCQ format. The major advantage over MCQs is that the larger number of response options reduces the likelihood that the question will cue the student to the correct answer; students also are less likely to recognize the correct answer. In many ways, the strengths and limitations of extended-matching questions are similar to those of multiple-choice questions.

Extended matching questions are organized around themes, and include multiple response options, instructions and a series of stems. Here is an example:

Theme:	Endocrine glands and hormones		
Options	A. Luteinizing hormone	E. Estrogen	I. Norepinephrine
	B. Vasopressin	F. Insulin	J. Prolactin
	C. Calcitonin	G. Testosterone	K. Oxytocin
	D. Glucagon	H. Melatonin	L. Progesterone
Instructions	For each statement below, select one hormone that best fits the description		
Stems	1. Secreted by the thyroid gland		
	2. Stimulates ovulation and corpus luteum formation		
	3. Lowers blood sugar		
	4. Secreted by pineal gland		

Strengths

- This question format can be used to construct an exam covering a wide range of content.
- This question format can be used to test knowledge recall as well as knowledge application.
- Scoring is highly reliable and objective, and like MCQs can easily be automated for efficiency.
- This question format is often used to test recall of factual information; there is less of a chance of students recognizing or guessing the right answer compared to MCQs. They can also be used to test problem-solving skills such as clinical diagnosis or patient management.

Limitations

- As with MCQs, time and practice are needed to write good questions that take advantage of the strengths of this format but do not cue the respondent.
- Similar to MCQs, these questions provide only minimal feedback to students to enhance their learning. Some examination software applications allow additional feedback either during or following the examination.

Reliability and Validity

- Like MCQs, this item format has high reliability because of the consistency of scoring over time or across examiners.
- The validity of an exam using extended matching questions is based on the representativeness of the test content compared to the instructional content. Like MCQs, questions derived from a test blueprint can assure a fair test in terms of content.

Construction Tips

- Extended matching questions are usually written around a theme. When the theme is based on a clinical scenario, research abstract or an image, the questions can require students to recall knowledge, interpret findings or suggest possible diagnoses.
- The response choices should be relatively brief, with the major content elements included in the questions.
- Avoid questions worded with negatives or double negatives.
- Avoid the use of response options that are irrelevant or silly.

There is an excellent resource for extended-matching questions available free-of-charge from the National Board of Medical Examiners website (www.nbme.org). Under publications, look for "Item Writing Manual: Constructing Written Test Questions for the Basic and Clinical Sciences" by Susan Case and David Swanson (2002).

Essays and Modified Essay Questions

These types of questions are characterized by the requirement that the student constructs a response rather than choose a correct response from the options provided. Essay and modified essay questions provide an opportunity to assess students' ability to apply knowledge to solve problems, organize ideas or information, and synthesize information (Cashin 1987). A sample essay question might be,

You are treating Sandy, a 57 year old woman who was diagnosed 6 months ago with Stage 2 adenocarcinoma of the right lung. Until a few days ago, her pain has been well-controlled. You have reevaluated the pain control and decided to initiate treatment with sustained release oral morphine. Sandy's brother is coming to the next appointment; he has concerns that his sister will become addicted to the pain medication. What will you say to Sandy's brother?

Modified essay questions are an assessment format that addresses some of the limitations of the essay question. A modified essay question is made up of one or more short answer questions. The student is provided with basic science or clinical information and then asked to write brief responses to one or more questions. When a series of questions is presented, additional information about the original problem can be provided at each subsequent step, guiding the students through an analytical process.

David is a 26 year old computer programmer, who lives alone with his dog Max. He has come to your office complaining of a persistent cough.

1. What are three likely diagnoses?
   a.
   b.
   c.
2. List five specific questions that would help you distinguish among these possibilities.
   a.
   b.
   c.
   d.
   e.

David tells you that the cough started about 5 days ago, and that many people in his office have called in sick lately. He has felt feverish and had some chills yesterday evening. He has been coughing up a small amount of thick green sputum.

3. List two diagnostic tests appropriate for work-up of this case.
   a.
   b.

Strengths

- This question format can be used to test written communication skills.
- Essay questions can focus on content related to knowledge or attitudes.
- Essay questions are best used to assess depth of knowledge within a limited area of content.
- This question format is familiar to students, and fairly straightforward for faculty to construct.
- Essay and modified essay questions are well-suited for formative feedback, since students can be provided with a model answer to help them understand their performance and prepare for future assessments.
- Modified essay questions require less time to score than traditional essay questions. Because student responses tend to be shorter and more succinct, these types of questions are less subject to scoring bias and can provide broader content

coverage, both of which increase the reliability and validity of the assessment. While essay questions can be used to assess higher levels of student cognitive ability, modified essay questions are ideal for testing knowledge recall that is not based on recognizing the correct answer as in MCQs.

Limitations

- Reliability is a major concern and there is a need to assure consistency of scoring over time and when multiple individuals are involved in scoring. Scoring of written responses is more likely to be affected by general subjective biases of the scorer, often referred to as halo effects. In practice halo effects occur when there is a possibility of giving some students the benefit of the doubt more often than other students when scoring written responses. An example might be students who are known to be strong performers or students who have done well on other parts of the assessment might be given the benefit of the doubt more often compared to weaker performers. The possibility of halo effects is more likely when student identities are known to scorers or when a single scorer is used.
- More time is required for scoring these responses than other formats.
- Tests based on essay-type questions are more limited in their content coverage because of the length of time required for students to respond to the questions as well as the length of time required for scoring.
- Essay questions require at least minimal written communication skills, and if communication skills are not the focus of the assessment, a lack of communication skills might limit a student's ability to achieve a high score even if they know the content.

Reliability and Validity

- Reliability is a major concern with these types of questions. The individuals scoring written responses might need to make some inferences about what the respondent meant to write because of poor written communication skills including organization, grammar and vocabulary, or due to vague wording. The opportunity for inference tends to reduce reliability.
- Reliability can be increased by having a clear scoring scheme developed prior to grading the questions. One approach would be to create a model answer and then allocate points to specific features of the answer, such as mentioning specific key content, presentation of a logical argument, recognition of a counter-argument or alternative explanations, or whatever else is appropriate to the question. When possible, all of the answers to one question should be scored at the same time, by the same person. If multiple people are scoring the exam, then each should grade all of the responses to a single question. Each essay question or set of modified essay questions should be graded independently of the other questions, and when possible the identity of the students should be unknown to the person grading the question to reduce the likelihood of bias.
- To create a test with high validity, it is important to make sure that the essay questions address important content as indicated by the course objectives and

overall course plan. Having several content experts review the model answer to each question can strengthen the validity of the assessment. This is particularly true when the question asks students to integrate concepts from across several content domains, which might not have been taught by the same instructor.

Construction Tips

- Write questions that outline a specific task for the students. Asking students to discuss a content area is not as clear or helpful as asking students to compare and contrast, describe, provide a justification or explain.
- To improve reliability and the sampling of course content, it is more effective to use a large number of modified essay questions requiring short answers than to use a more limited number of essay questions requiring long written answers.
- Prepare a model answer after constructing the test question. This helps to increase scoring consistency by assuring that the answer you expect is reasonable given the question, and clarifies how points are assigned to content and presentation of the answer.
- To reduce bias and improve consistency, score only one essay question or set of modified essay questions at a time, and if feasible have separate scorers for each essay question. When this is not possible, rescoring a small set of answers can help maintain consistency. The subset of rescored answers should be sampled from throughout the set of examinations to make sure that the application of the scoring criteria did not change over time.
- When possible, score the answers to the questions with the identity of the students anonymous to the scorer.
- When used for formative assessment, student learning can be enhanced by providing students with a model answer as well as feedback about common errors observed when scoring.

Short Answer Questions

Short answer questions require students to provide brief answers to questions. The responses usually require only one or two words or a brief phrase. Short answer questions are sometimes presented as fill-in-the-blank questions.

1. A middle-aged financial planner presents with a several month history of stomach discomfort. He has found limited relief with over-the-counter antacids, although these are now less effective than before. His discomfort is aggravated by caffeine, alcohol and late night snacking. What is the likely differential diagnosis for this patient?
2. In planning the diagnostic work-up for this patient, list two tests you would definitely include to aid in your diagnosis.

Like essay questions, short answer questions require students to provide a response rather than choose or recognize a response from list of possibilities provided. However, because short answer questions require briefer responses, more questions can be included within an exam, achieving greater content coverage than with essay questions (Rademaker et al., 2005).

Strengths

- High content coverage is possible.
- This format of question is familiar to students.
- This question format has high reliability and validity.
- Faculty find it relatively easy to construct short answer questions.

Limitations

- These types of questions tend to focus on knowledge, and are used to test knowledge recall and comprehension rather than higher level abilities.
- Scored questions indicating the correct answers provide limited feedback to students to improve learning.
- Scoring cannot easily be automated: this question format requires more time to score than MCQs but less time than essay or modified essay questions.

Reliability and Validity

- Reliability can be achieved by writing questions that are clear to the student. Also important are clearly written model answers to each question. The distribution of points for the responses should be clearly specified. While bias is less likely to apply to scoring short answer questions, the likelihood of halo effects can be minimized by the same procedures described for essay and modified essay questions.
- Using a blueprint to create short answer questions that representatively sample from the course objectives and content is important. As mentioned previously, having several content experts review the model answers can strengthen the validity of the assessment. This is particularly true when there might be multiple possible correct answers for a question, or when the correct answer can be described in multiple ways.

Construction Tips

- Write questions that are clear and specific.
- Prepare the short answer questions and the model answers at the same time. Afterwards, reread the questions and answers again to assure that the expected answer is reasonable given the question.
- To reduce bias and improve consistency, score the all the answers to a single set of questions at the same time. Rescoring a small subset of answers can help maintain consistency throughout the scoring process.
- Score the answers to the questions with the identity of the students anonymous if possible.

Faculty Global Ratings

Faculty global ratings can be used to summarize impressions of overall performance within a defined situation such as a clinical encounter or assignment involving teamwork. Global ratings can be aggregated over time to represent typical behavior in vital situations, such as a clinical rotation or small group setting (Gray 1996). Global ratings are based on a number of important domains of performance or behavior, with a judgment of the extent to which desired performance was observed.

---

1. Rate the student's ability to obtain information about the presenting problem in this simulated clinical encounter

   a. Obtained little or no information
   b. Obtained some information, but with major omissions or errors
   c. Obtained most information indicative of satisfactory performance
   d. Obtained most or all information with thorough exploration of patient problem

2. Rate the student's participation in your small group discussion section with regards to his/her ability to display respect

a. Below expectations	displays disdain for other group members or their opinions; interrupts group members or preceptor
b. At expectations	engages in group discussions without conveying disrespect; avoids interrupting group members
c. Exceeds expectations	seeks out alternative points of view; self-monitors own participation so that others can contribute

---

Strengths

- Global ratings by faculty tend to have high validity when they are based on the observation of behaviors of interest within a real or simulated context.
- This format can be used to assess general categories of performance such as clinical skills, problem-solving, teamwork, presentation skills and professionalism; participation and preparation in a small group learning context such as problem-based learning; or achievement of course objectives when used to rate group presentations or other assignments.
- This format is useful in formative assessment to provide learner feedback.

Limitations

- Reliability can be variable when there are differences in expectations and standards among faculty providing the ratings. Training and practice can reduce variability across faculty raters.
- Faculty need to set aside time to observe students prior to completing the global ratings.
- Halo effects and other subjective biases are common.

Reliability and Validity

- Specific training and practice is needed to achieve standardization (Holmboe et al., 2004): consensus among faculty raters as to the rating categories and expectations for the ratings within a category. The rating form should have specific descriptions of the expected behaviors for each of the rating points within a category. To limit the impact of halo effects and other subjective biases, the use of multiple raters and multiple rating sessions is recommended.
- Validity is evident from the behaviors sampled on the rating form. Expert faculty can be used to determine those behaviors that represent the target performance in the learning context (e.g., PBL group, clerkship, etc.) where the form will be used.

Construction Tips

- The rating form should only include observable behaviors; these behaviors should occur at a frequency that makes them readily observable.
- Some people are better raters than others, depending on the rating task. Over time, it might be evident that some raters are more reliable than others. Using individuals who are reliable will improve the usefulness of the data obtained from the rating form for feedback and student performance decisions.
- The rating form should have specific descriptions of the expected behaviors for each of the rating points within a category.
- Halo effects and other subjective biases can be reduced through the use of multiple raters and multiple rating sessions.
- Student learning can be enhanced by providing students with copies of the rating forms to be used for assessment, indicating the categories of performance and the expected performance within each category.

Faculty Checklist Ratings

Global ratings as discussed above are frequently based on assigning scores on a multi-point rating scale for each of a variety of behaviors. In contrast, checklist ratings of direct observations are based on checklists that indicate the presence or absence of a specific behavior or the component parts of a complex behavior.

Please rate this student's performance of the following portions of the neurologic exam			
	Done correctly	Done incorrectly	Not done
1. Motor			
a. Strength of arms	1	2	3
b. Arms outstretched, eyes closed	1	2	3
c. Strength of legs	1	2	3
2. Reflexes			
a. Biceps (inside of elbow)	1	2	3
b. Triceps (back of arm at elbow)	1	2	3
c. Brachioradialis (wrist/forearm)	1	2	3
d. Patellar (knee)	1	2	3
e. Achilles (ankle)	1	2	3

Strengths

- Checklist ratings tend to have high validity because they are based on direct observation of specific behaviors of interest. The checklist represents a list of the specific skills expected of students.
- Checklist ratings can be used to assess specific skill sets such as clinical skills related to communication, history-taking, physical examination, or presentation skills related to a class project or clinical case.
- Checklist ratings provide specific feedback to learners about the elements of their performance judged to be present or absent.

Limitations

- Rater factors such as poor standardization, inconsistent expectations, and halo effects can reduce the reliability of the assessments.
- A limitation of rating forms is that for rating purposes, target skills are broken down into essential elements. While this approach is appropriate and helpful for students learning a new skill, it is less appropriate for assessing the performance of more experienced students or practitioners.

Reliability and Validity

- Reliability can be improved by having clearly defined checklist items, and raters familiar with the skills to be rated. The less inference required of raters when completing the checklist, the greater the likelihood of reliable ratings. This also reduces the likelihood of halo effects.
- Validity is high for this approach because the rating forms are based on specific target behaviors, often broken down into essential elements. For students learning new skills, this can provide feedback about specific components that were omitted or incorrectly executed. The items on the rating form can be based on the list of steps used to teach the skill.
- More advanced students and practitioners, with practice, will move beyond step-by-step performance of skills as they were initially learned to more integrated performance. More advanced learners are less likely to repeat the key elements in a rote fashion while still effectively performing the desired task. For this reason, when assessing the skills of advanced learners, global ratings might be more appropriate than checklists.

Construction Tips

- Reliability is improved when the number of options for each checklist item is limited. Frequently checklists are constructed with paired options for each item on the checklist, such as done/not done, observed/not observed, or satisfactory/unsatisfactory. Sometimes a third option is included indicating that a step was attempted: (1) done correctly, (2) done incorrectly (3) not done. This format can be used when the student attempts a skill unsuccessfully, and there is reason to distinguish this from skills not attempted, such as when the rating form is used for formative feedback to students.

- If the checklist ratings are to be performed from memory, such as might occur when a standardized patient completes the checklist after a simulated encounter with a student, the number of total items on the checklist should be limited to what can reasonably be remembered by the rater (Wallace 2007).

Oral Examinations

An oral examination requires students to answer a series of preselected questions; these are typically based on standard stimulus information such as a patient case. For example, based on the patient information provided, the examiner can ask questions about differential diagnoses, pertinent missing data, additional testing, patient management as well as clinical reasoning, data interpretation or basic science content underlying the student's responses (Mancall and Bashook 1995). The length of time per case can vary depending on whether breadth or depth of understanding is desirable, as well as whether the exam is being used for formative or summative assessment.

> David is a 26 year old computer programmer, who lives alone with his dog Max. He has come to your office complaining of a persistent cough.
>
> 1. List three diagnoses that you would include in your differential diagnosis.
> 2. List five specific questions that would help you distinguish among these possibilities.
> 3. List two diagnostic tests appropriate for work-up of this case.
>   a. What is the rationale for each?

Strengths

- Oral exams can be used to assess knowledge and attitudes.
- This assessment format can be used to assess higher order clinical problem-solving such as application and synthesis of knowledge, ability to prioritize features of a patient case and evaluate treatment options.
- Oral exams provide insights into students' organizational and verbal skills.
- When used in formative settings, oral exams can be used to provide students with immediate feedback and provide instructors with information about students' approaches to problem-solving and reasoning.

Limitations

- Reliability can be problematic as a result of rater factors such as poor standardization, inconsistent expectations, and halo effects.
- Like essay exams, oral exams provide limited coverage of content and cases, which can limit the validity of the assessment.

- Oral exams require verbal and language skills, which can limit students' ability to communicate their content knowledge.
- This assessment format is not familiar to many students, which increases their anxiety.
- Time is required for scoring the results of an oral exam, particularly when a large number of examiners is involved.

Reliability and Validity

- Significant training of the examiners is required for reliability to be achieved. The training must address performance expectations and standards, as well as the use of structured rating forms to record student performance. The use of multiple examiners is recommended to reduce halo effects and other rater biases.
- Because oral examinations are limited in the amount of content that can be covered, longer exams are more valid than shorter exams. It is also important that the exam is standardized in terms of the content to be covered and the specific rating forms for scoring each examinee.

Construction Tips

- An effective strategy to improve reliability is the use of paired or tripled examiners for each question. Thus each student will have a different group of raters for each oral exam question. Each examiner should grade or rate the examinees independently.
- To improve the validity of this exam, the selection of the cases to be covered should focus on important content; longer exams are more valid than shorter exams because of the increase in content coverage.
- When cases are used as the stimulus for the oral exam, the same cases and questions should be used for all examinees to maintain standardization. However the order of questions can be varied across examinees.
- As with essay exams, model answers and explicit grading criteria for each question should be developed prior to the oral exam. All raters should be familiar with the grading criteria and rating form.

Standardized Patients and OSCEs

Standardized patients are actual patients or laypeople trained to portray a patient for teaching and/or assessment purposes. The standardized patient can provide a stimulus to assess a student's skills related to communications, history-taking or physical examination. As the term suggests, standardized patients are used in assessment to provide a standard clinical encounter against which to judge student performance.

Standardized patients are typically used as part of an objective standardized clinical examination (OSCE) (Hardin and Gleeson 1979). An OSCE provides an opportunity to assess student knowledge and skills that are not easily assessed using more traditional paper and pencil-based examinations. This assessment format involves students moving through a series of clinical encounters, with each one requiring specific tasks. Skills related to communications, history-taking, physical examination and written records are typically a part of an OSCE. A typical OSCE might be made up of six to twelve stations, each involving a 15-min encounter with a standardized patient, with 10 min afterwards to complete a written record or answer specific knowledge or interpretation questions about the case. In each of these situations, student performance is judged using the methods described above under checklists, rating forms, essay and oral exams. The Medical Council of Canada and the National Board of Medical Examiners both have implemented an OSCE as part of their licensure process.

Strengths

- Simulated encounters provide a realistic yet safe context for assessing student performance of basic clinical skills as well as more integrated performance required in complex clinical encounters, such as deriving differential diagnoses, treatment planning and documenting clinical findings. The complexity of the encounters can be varied to accommodate the experience of the learners.
- Simulated encounters can provide students with immediate feedback about their performance. Alternatively they can be recorded for later review and critique. This review can involve students and faculty reviewing the recordings together, or can be completed by the student independently as a self-assessment.
- Simulated encounters can be customized to focus on educational goals and values important to the institution.

Limitations

- Despite the high fidelity of the approach, it does require some suspension of belief on the part of students.
- Simulated encounters are resource intensive in terms of time, case development, raters and standardized patients.
- This format is unfamiliar to students and initially can cause anxiety, especially when used for summative assessment.

Reliability and Validity

- Reliability and validity increase with the length of the OSCE. Adding more cases or stations increases content coverage and improves validity. To accomplish this, the length of each station might be reduced to shorten the overall testing time per student. However, as the time per encounter decreases, the fidelity of the encounter might be reduced.
- In rating the performance of students during the encounters, checklists and global rating forms are frequently used. Each has their own strengths and limitations with regards to reliability and validity that must be addressed.

Construction Tips

- The formative use of simulated encounters is a very powerful technique and can provide students with tangible feedback to improve performance. In formative settings students often value this approach to assessment.
- The checklists to record student performance during a simulated encounter should be only as long as necessary. When completed from memory as is often the case when used by standardized patients, the value of long checklists and rating forms is limited by patients' ability to remember the specifics of the encounter.

Technology-Based Simulations

Technology-based simulations for performance assessment provide standardized conditions for studying and assessing clinical performance. Through the use of mannequins, computers, artificial limbs, virtual reality and other tools, simulations can be created for assessment purposes that provide a realistic challenge to students based on a clinical problem (Tekian et al., 1999). The advantage of this format is that there is no danger to patients, and depending on how they are implemented the simulations can provide instant feedback. Written and computer-based simulations have been used to assess clinical reasoning, diagnostic plans and management. Simulators can be used alone or in conjunction with standardized patients. Additional information about this format is found in Chap. 8.

Strengths

- Technology-based simulations are particularly well-suited for assessing procedural skills, critical care decision-making and teamwork.
- When observed by faculty, this approach can be a powerful tool for improving instruction and providing feedback to students.
- This type of simulation provides important skill-focused training in a context that does not jeopardize patient safety.
- Technology-based simulations are useful for both formative and summative assessment.

Limitations

- Technology-based simulations are less realistic than standardized patient encounters, but can provide opportunities to demonstrate skills that might be impractical, uncomfortable or embarrassing for standardized patients.
- Simulator technology often is expensive.

Reliability and Validity

- Technology–based simulations create highly standardized test situations for students. Some simulators collect response data and provide quantitative feedback. This tends to be reliable and valid. To the extent that performance is judged on the basis of checklists or rating scales, these approaches each have strengths and weaknesses, which have previously been discussed.

Construction Tips

- A complete discussion of the effective use of simulators can be found in Chap. 8.

Peer Assessments

Peer assessment is usually implemented using global rating forms; respondents are asked to rate a student's performance on specific criteria or to indicate the relative frequency of specific target behaviors. Alternatively, respondents could be asked to divide a total number of points (e.g., 100 points) among all of the members of a small group, and provide a reason for the number of points awarded to each person. Peer assessments are useful in that they provide feedback from multiple sources about an individual's performance. The feedback to a student can be the aggregated scores across multiple peer raters. In addition, the ratings can be aggregated across a variety of situations or encounters.

For each of the attributes listed below, please rate the performance of this student compared to other students in your small group					
	Well below average	Average			Well above average
1. Preparation for small group sessions	1	2	3	4	5
2. Participation in group discussions	1	2	3	4	5
3. Leadership during group discussions	1	2	3	4	5
4. Encouragement of contributions from others	1	2	3	4	5
5. Respectful of other points of view	1	2	3	4	5
6. Contribution to group assignments	1	2	3	4	5

Strengths

- This format is most appropriate for observable behaviors and skills.
- Peer assessments can provide insights into professional behavior and teamwork, which are often difficult to assess using other methods.
- Peer assessments provide a credible source of performance information related to daily observable behaviors. This is especially useful for formative feedback when provided in a timely and confidential manner.
- Participation in peer assessments provides students with valuable experience in giving and receiving feedback. It also provides students with an opportunity to systematically compare their own performance with the performance of others within a similar context.

Limitations

- Peer assessments can be provided through the use of rating checklists, global ratings or written narratives. Each of these methods has inherent limitations that have already been described.
- A general lack of familiarity with this approach is threatening to students.
- Some evaluators, especially peers, might be reluctant to provide negative feedback to their fellow students.
- Data collection, analysis and feedback can be cumbersome when used for assessing many individuals.
- A supportive learning environment is essential. When confidentiality and trust are not safeguarded, the validity of the data collected and the value of the feedback to students is significantly diminished. In the worst case scenario, peer assessments can be experienced by students as threatening, critical and hurtful.

Reliability and Validity

- A large number of respondents are required to obtain reliable ratings: nurses have been found to be reliable raters while patients and faculty are less reliable, which requires more ratings. This is particularly important when this approach is used for high stakes outcomes such as recertification. Individuals chosen to provide ratings should have multiple opportunities to observe the behavior of the student in question.
- Validity is a function of the process used to develop the rating form, the individuals from whom ratings are obtained, and the length of time over which raters have observed the target behaviors.

Construction Tips

- Students should know the rating categories used in the peer assessment in advance so the process is transparent and less threatening.
- It is helpful to provide guidelines and examples about giving feedback to others so that the feedback is constructive and appropriate for the expected level of performance.
- The quality of the feedback will improve over time with practice; this is especially true for students, who frequently have little experience with this form of assessment.
- Peer assessments can be implemented as part of a 360° assessment (Raksha et al., 2004), which involves ratings-based assessment of an individual's behavior. The ratings are completed by a wide range of others who have contact with the individual. In a clinical setting, this frequently includes peers, supervisors, instructors, nursing staff and allied health personnel; in some cases patients might be included.
- Peer assessment can focus on skills related to interpersonal and written communication, professionalism, teamwork and leadership.
- Although most frequently used in clinical settings to evaluate student performance, this type of assessment can be used in small group instruction, clinical skills training and other settings.

Self-Assessments

Self-assessment is often an informal process for students as they progress through their education. There are relatively few opportunities for students to use structured self-assessment for formative assessment; for a variety of reasons, some of which are obvious, the use of self-assessment for summative progress decisions is even rarer. The actual format of self-assessments can be written or based on rating forms, focusing on global attributes. Self-assessments are probably most valuable when used in conjunction with similar assessments from other sources such as peers or teachers.

Strengths

- Self-assessment provides students with a valuable opportunity to become more critical of their own performance as well as to develop insight and responsibility for their performance.
- Self-assessment provides a setting for reflection and creation of a self-initiated plan for personal and professional development.
- This approach can be used to self-assess strengths and limitations related to knowledge, clinical skills and personal attitudes.
- Because the assessment is self-generated, it provides a unique perspective on students' abilities, particularly when used with other information to provide formative feedback.
- The structure and content of the self-assessment form can be used to direct the scope of the self-assessment.

Limitations

- The most significant limitation of self-assessment is our own difficulty of seeing ourselves as others see us. This makes self-assessment a challenging task for many to do well, and even with experience, our inherent limitations in self-monitoring restrict the application of this approach.
- Since rating scales are typically the format used for self-assessment, the limitations associated with that technique apply to self-assessment.
- Students' lack of familiarity with a systematic approach to self-assessment makes this form of assessment threatening for many students.
- This approach is best used within the context of a supportive learning environment, where students feel safe to reveal their own limitations and confidentiality is assured.

Reliability and Validity

- Reliability can be increased by clearly specifying the self-assessment rating task in terms of the behaviors to be rated, the time period covered by the assessment, and well-defined criteria and standards to guide the assessment.
- Using explicit criteria for structuring the assessment, acknowledged and endorsed by students and faculty, will enhance the validity of the self-assessment ratings.

Construction Tips

- The rating form used to guide student self-assessment should focus on specific behaviors and outcomes, e.g., what was tried and/or accomplished.
- To promote broad support and endorsement of the self-assessment rating scheme, open discussions involving students and faculty can be used to delineate the criteria for judging performance as well as elicit possible standards for each criterion related to satisfactory and unsatisfactory performance.
- This form of assessment can be combined with peer and faculty assessments to provide multisource feedback. This approach also helps balance unrealistic self-appraisals (Fitzgerald et al., 2003).

Portfolios

A portfolio is a collection of evidence organized around specific themes as a means of assessing knowledge skills and attitudes (Buckley et al., 2009; Challis 1999). The major components of a portfolio include a statement of purpose for the portfolio, examples of evidence selected by the student to document performance, as well as a reflective statement by the student regarding the portfolio content. A portfolio also can be a journal or educational diary chronicling learner experiences and insights over time, beginning or ending with a reflective self-assessment of the assembled experiences.

Strengths

- The task of selecting representative evidence of achievement provides an opportunity for reflection and self-appraisal.
- A wide range of evidence can be included in a portfolio including written documents and projects, letters of appreciation or recognition, presentations, digital media and resources, citations, logbooks of patient encounters, assessment results, reflective self-assessments and survey results.
- The assembled evidence provides insight into the learner's ability to apply their knowledge and skills in integrative tasks, as well as the growth of their knowledge and abilities over time.
- Central to most portfolios is an integrative reflective essay that provides insight into higher level cognitive abilities as well as the learner's own ability to self-assess their achievements and what has been learned.
- Portfolios can be used for formative or summative assessment, and can be an important source of information when combined with faculty mentorship.
- Portfolios can also be used for summative assessment such as faculty promotion decisions.

Limitations

- The task of selecting, organizing and interpreting the representative evidence of achievement is time consuming.

- Presumably the examples selected for inclusion in the portfolio are the best evidence the learner has of their performance, and therefore only a selective sample of performance is presented.
- This format is unfamiliar to many students and faculty, both in terms of putting a portfolio together and making judgments from a portfolio.

Reliability and Validity

- As with other forms of assessment, clear specification of the purpose and content of the portfolio is important to assure validity. The relationship of the portfolio to learning objectives or promotion criteria enhances validity. Clear instructions can help define the types of evidence appropriate for inclusion, the number of examples to include, and the content of the reflective essay.
- Reliability is achieved through the use of multiple ratings of the portfolio content, as well as the use of multiple forms of evidence included in the portfolio to demonstrate specific educational outcomes or performance.
- Also important is an understanding by students and raters of the criteria by which the portfolio will be judged as well as the rating form, derived from these criteria, which will be used as a basis for the judgments.
- Because the assessment of the portfolio is ultimately made through the use of rating forms, the issues associated with the reliability and validity of rating forms also have bearing here.

Construction tips

- Providing learners with the responsibility to meaningfully choose the evidence to include in the portfolio enhances their ownership of the portfolio. Another way of promoting ownership is involving students in the discussion of how the portfolios will be evaluated: the criteria and standards to be used.
- Portfolios can include a wide range of evidence such as: abstracts or brief descriptions of research or educational projects; publications or presentations; case studies; self- or peer-assessments; awards and letters of recognition or appreciation documenting learner achievements; letters or documents describing service contributions to professional or community organizations; awards; materials from websites or digital media that have been developed; personal reflections on specific achievements, activities, ethical dilemmas, challenging patients, etc. Almost any type of evidence might have value in a portfolio depending on its purpose.
- Software tools have been developed to assist in the compilation of evidence into an electronic portfolio. These tools range from blogs, wikis, online learning management systems to specific portfolio systems. See Chap. 10 for more information.
- Criteria for judging the content of a portfolio often focuses on the student's reflective essay regarding the achievements represented by the assembled evidence. The evidence can also be interpreted in terms of the breadth and depth of content; comparison of different types of content; and areas of strength, weakness or achievement not represented within the portfolio. Another use of the portfolio is as a stimulus for discussion between students and instructors or mentors.

- An assessment derived from a portfolio can focus on the skills, knowledge or attitudes in judgments of the technical achievements represented by the evidence, as well as the application of theory or the ethics and values inherent in the content.
- There are circumstances when standard criteria for assessing portfolios might not be desirable, such as when the portfolio is implemented as a means of documenting the achievements and progress made by individuals as part of an individualized educational plan for independent study or remediation.

Reporting and Feedback

Feedback to Students

As mentioned earlier in this chapter, an important consequence of assessment is that students receive feedback about their learning. Many of the assessment methods described in this chapter will be used for summative assessment, providing reliable and valid information from which student progress decisions can be made. Some of these assessments are also well-suited for providing students with detailed information about their strengths as well as areas for improvement. It is this level of detail in the feedback to students that provides them with the greatest opportunities for learning from their assessment experiences and building confidence in their abilities. Formative feedback is also important for building confidence and reducing anxiety when students are confronted with forms of assessment that are unfamiliar to them.

Depending on the assessment, feedback can take the form of detailed model performance such as model answers for essay and oral exams, videos of expected skill performance, sample portfolios and the like. Other forms of feedback include summaries of the most common errors made by students during an assessment, and information about why a specific response choice was right or wrong. Of course, written comments related to the students' specific responses are very helpful but can be very time consuming. Another strategy is to have students self-assess their performance as a means of comparison with instructor feedback. To optimize the value of assessments as feedback experience for students:

- use clear criteria for grading performance
- provide feedback in a timely manner
- include both positive and negative feedback when practical
- make feedback as specific as possible

Feedback to Faculty

It is important that aggregated student performance information be available to the medical school committees responsible for oversight of the curriculum. Aggregate performance information can be used to provide evidence of the success of new programs, curricula or modes of instruction. Another important use of aggregated student performance data is to provide valid evidence for decision-making and supplements the perceptions of students or faculty. It provides a systematic approach to data collection that can be used to answer specific questions about effectiveness and outcomes, and perhaps give rise to further questions about the curriculum. Such evidence can be crucial in the face of personal testimonials or opinions derived from one person's experience with a specific student or educational experience. This information can be part of an ongoing effort to monitor an educational program or diagnose curricular problems as part of a systematic program review. See Chap. 16 for more information.

References

Amin Z, Seng CY, Eng KH (2006) Practical guide to medical student assessment. World Scientific Publishing Company, Singapore

Anderson L, Krathwohl D (eds) (2001) A taxonomy for learning, teaching, and assessing: a revision of Bloom's taxonomy of educational objectives. Longman, New York

Buckley S, Coleman J, Davison I, Khan K, Zamora J (2009) The educational effects of portfolios on undergraduate student learning: a Best Evidence Medical Education (BEME) systematic review. BEME Guide No. 11. Med Teach 31:282–298

Case S, Swanson D (2002) Constructing written test questions for the basic and clinical sciences, Third edition (revised). National Board of Medical Examiners. Available at: http://www.nbme.org/pdf/itemwriting_2003/2003iwgwhole.pdf

Cashin W (1987) iDEA Paper #17: Improving essay tests. The iDEA Center, Center for Faculty Evaluation and Development, Kansas State University. Available from:http://www.theideacenter.org/sites/default/files/Idea_Paper_17.pdf

Challis M (1999) AMEE medical education guide no. 11 (revised): portfolio-based learning and assessment in medical education. Med Teach 21:370–386

Cook D, Beckman T (2006) Current concepts in validity and reliability for psychometric instruments: theory and application. Am J Med 119:166.e7–166.e16

Epstein R, Hundert E (2002) Defining and assessing professional competence. J Am Med Assoc 287(2):226–235

Fitzgerald J, White C, Gruppen L (2003) A longitudinal study of self-assessment accuracy. Med Educ 37(7):645–649

Gray J (1996) Global rating scales in residency education. Acad Med 71:S55–S63

Hardin R, Gleeson F (1979) Assessment of medical competence using an objective structured clinical examination (OSCE). Med Educ 13(1):41–54

Holmboe E, Hawkins R, Huot S (2004) Effects of training in direct observation of medical residents' clinical competence: a randomized trial. Ann Intern Med 140(11):874–881

Mancall EL, Bashook PG (eds) (1995) Assessing clinical reasoning: the oral examination and alternative methods. American Board of Medical Specialties, Evanston

Mehrens WA, Lehmann IJ (1991) Measurement and evaluation in education and psychology, 4th edn. Holt, Rinehart and Winston, Fort Worth

Miller G (1990) The assessment of clinical skills/competence/performance. Acad Med 65(9):S63–S67

Miller AH, Imrie BW, Cox K (1998) Student assessment in higher education. In: A handbook for assessing performance. Kogan Page, London

Rademaker J, ten Cate T, Bar P (2005) Progress testing with short answer questions. Med Teach 27(7):578–582

Raksha J, Ling F, Jaeger J (2004) Assessment of a 360-degree instrument to evaluate residents' competency in interpersonal and communication skills. Acad Med 79(5):458–463

Sepdham D, Julka M, Hofmann J, Dobbie A (2007) Using the RIME model for learner assessment and feedback. Fam Med 39(3):161–163

Shumway J, Harden R (2003) AMEE Guide No. 25: the assessment of learning outcomes for the competent and reflective physician. Med Teach 25(6):569–584

Tekian A, McGuire C, McGaghie W (eds) (1999) Innovative simulations for assessing professional competence. University of Illinois Press, Chicago

Wallace P (2007) Coaching standardized patients. Springer, New York

Chapter 16
Documenting the Trajectory of Your Teaching

Nicole K. Roberts

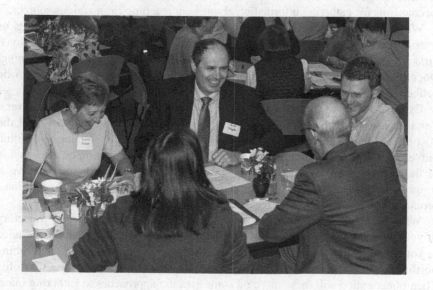

Abstract Being a teacher in a medical school is a challenge. It's a delightful, rewarding, surprising, engaging, inspiring honor of a challenge, but a challenge nonetheless. Whether you give lectures to large groups, facilitate small groups, guide teams in Team-Based Learning, or teach in clinical rounds, you are likely to find that as you try things out, you learn more and more about what does and does not work. The changes you make, for better or worse, plot the trajectory of your

N.K. Roberts, Ph.D. (✉)
The Academy for Scholarship in Education, Department of Medical Education,
Southern Illinois University School of Medicine, Springfield, IL,
PO Box 19681, 62794, USA
e-mail: nroberts@siumed.edu

K.N. Huggett and W.B. Jeffries (eds.), *An Introduction to Medical Teaching*,
DOI 10.1007/978-94-017-9066-6_16, © Springer Science+Business Media Dordrecht 2014

teaching—the ascent of a successful lecture, the descent of a difficult tutor group, the subsequent correction in style or approach that demonstrates your reflection on feedback or evaluation. This chapter encourages you to be deliberate and evidence-based in your approach to improving your teaching. In this chapter, we will encourage you to document the trajectory of your teaching, and will discuss mechanisms for gathering information about your teaching from various sources.

Introduction

Chapter 17 on the scholarship of teaching encourages you to be deliberate and evidence-based in your approach to improving your teaching. In this chapter, we will encourage you to document the trajectory of your teaching, and will discuss mechanisms for gathering information about your teaching from various sources.

Why go through the trouble of collecting information about your teaching, or considering how you have changed over the years? There are several reasons. First, there is the satisfaction derived from observing your own growth and learning. Documentation can facilitate your ability to reflect on your practice and to be deliberate in the changes you make.

External forces may also weigh on your decision to document your progress. For instance, with increasing frequency the public questions the cost, and the cost-effectiveness of higher education. Universities document their value, and within universities, individuals document their effectiveness in delivering on the mission of the university. For the teaching professor, this means not just being effective at research and service, but also being effective in teaching. In fact, in some institutions, promotion and tenure decisions rest on documented effectiveness of teaching.

What follows is a discussion of one mechanism for documenting the trajectory of your teaching, along with some thoughts about materials that might be included in your documentation. In this chapter, we will discuss the concept of the teaching portfolio. We will discuss potential content, uses, and structure of the portfolio. Then our attention will focus more on some specific approaches to gathering information that will be useful to the documentation of the trajectory of your teaching.

Portfolios

A portfolio is simply a mechanism to help you tell the story of your teaching to yourself and to others. It is a collection of materials, either paper or digital, that documents various aspects of your work as an educator. A portfolio can be used to demonstrate your effectiveness, show your growth over time, explain how you respond to feedback and evaluation, document your commitment to the teaching mission of your institution, and help you advocate for your promotion and/or tenure. Creating and maintaining an educational portfolio gives you cause to reflect on and refine your practice in a systematic fashion. It is also a method of communicating with others. You will likely share at least some aspects of your portfolio with a variety of audiences, including your supervisor, a trusted mentor, or a promotion and tenure committee.

Essential elements to the educator's portfolio include the following:

Educational philosophy statement: Your statement of your educational philosophy will likely change as you gain experience and knowledge of educational theory. However, it is useful to think about what matters to you as an educator. What do you think the educator's role is in student learning? The role of students? How do you make decisions about what to teach, and how to teach? It will be useful for you to revisit your educational philosophy periodically to see how experience has changed your assumptions.

Five-year goals as an educator: As with your educational philosophy, you may find that experience causes you to change your five year goals, however, creating the goal statement allows you to begin to solidify what you want to do as an educator. It also gives you a prism through which you can evaluate new opportunities and make rational decisions about whether or not to take them on.

Educational contributions in any or all of five activity categories

1. Teaching
2. Learner Assessment
3. Curriculum Development
4. Mentoring and Advising
5. Educational Leadership and Administration (Baldwin et al. 2008)

Simpson and colleagues suggest the Q^2 Engage standard for documenting any of these activities: Quantity, Quality, and Engagement with the educational community. To document quantity, you will collect information about the types and frequencies of education activities in which you engage. To document quality, you will collect information about the effectiveness and excellence of your educational activities. To demonstrate engagement with the educational community, you will collect evidence that your work was informed by what is known in the field of education, and that over time, you have contributed to the field. Of course, your documentation will also include a description of the activity and your role in it (Simpson et al. 2007).

When you document your educational contributions, you will likely collect all evidence of any of the categories listed. As you become more experienced, you will begin to evaluate materials, choosing those that do the best job of telling the story you intend to tell about your teaching.

For instance, you may wish to tell a story about how you are exceptionally responsive to learners' needs. To tell that story, you might begin with refining your educational philosophy to show why you value responsiveness to learner needs. In your philosophy, you might reflect on what in the educational literature suggests that responsiveness is useful and effective. Then you might review the instances of your teaching that were exceptionally effective in demonstrating your responsiveness to learner needs, and how you used a scholarly approach to developing your approaches to teaching—and so on for any of the other categories in which you made an educational contribution. As you continue your portfolio development, you'll want to refer also to Chap. 17.

For help structuring a portfolio, you can download a template created by the Educational Scholars Program of the Academic Pediatrics Association. This template provides a structure and some concrete guidance on how to construct your portfolio, and it can be adapted to suit your particular needs. The template can be found on MedEdPORTAL: https://www.mededportal.org/publication/626

Evaluation of Teaching

Some of the key elements of your portfolio will derive from evaluations of your teaching and evaluations of student learning. In this segment, we will discuss elements of evaluation, definitions and purposes of evaluative activities, how you might go about gathering evaluative material, and what you might do with the material once you've gathered it.

Definitions and Purposes of Evaluative Activities

Evaluative activities span a continuum, from feedback to formal summative evaluation. Here we will discuss each of these ways of gathering information about performance. In addition, we will define some important concepts related to evaluation.

Feedback is a source of formative information. It is the first source of information you might seek about your educational activities. Feedback can be formal or informal, but regardless, its purpose is to provide information about the successful or failing parts of a recent performance. The intention of feedback is to reinforce success and correct failures in order to improve subsequent performances.

Feedback might include information you infer from watching your learners. When they lean forward in their seats as you lecture, they are providing feedback that suggests that what you are saying is holding their interest. Conversely, when they put their heads down on their desks, they are giving you feedback that says you have lost the battle for their attention. When your audience buzzes about your topic, you infer their interest. When your audience thanks you, you infer they got what they wanted. Though this level of feedback may tell you *that* something is going well or poorly, it doesn't give you information about *why*. For information about what worked, what didn't, and why, you should be deliberate in seeking feedback.

You can request feedback from various sources. Logical sources include participants in your educational activity, a trusted mentor or colleague, or even a supervisor. If your school has a teaching academy, you could ask a member of the academy to observe you. You might ask somebody in advance to observe your educational activity and tell you how it went. You could ask them to observe for a particular element or portion to see if it was successful or not. You could ask for a simple description of your teaching. Or you might ask to be video recorded and to have an expert review your tape with you.

In order to assess whether or not your teaching encounter has served its purpose, you might ask participants to tell you (verbally or in writing) what they learned from the encounter, or what they are still unclear about, or what they wanted to learn but didn't.

It's important to understand, though, that the purpose of feedback is to guide your future performance. It is not to make a judgment about your quality as a teacher. Instead, it is intended to help the trajectory of your teaching ability rise, and to make corrections when it falls off. It will be useful for you to keep a record of the feedback you receive and your responses to it, to demonstrate your willingness and ability to reflect on your teaching practice.

Formative Evaluation

Like feedback, formative evaluation serves the purpose of helping you improve your educational efforts. It answers questions like "As of now, how are you doing, what is going well, and what should you try to improve?" It may be useful to think of formative evaluation as a mechanism to process and analyze feedback and to respond to it to ensure that your teaching continues to improve. Once again, there are several sources you might consult for formative evaluations. For instance, if you are teaching a formal class, you might distribute a questionnaire to your students in the middle of the semester asking them how the class is going thus far. If your teaching is primarily in the clinical setting, you might ask your students mid clerkship if they are getting what they want from the experience. You can use this information to adjust your teaching practices as needed.

Summative Evaluation

Summative evaluation is intended to provide a judgment about your teaching ability or your educational interventions. It is used to make a decision about a person or a program. Summative evaluations take place at the end of a given term, for instance, at the end of a semester or the end of a clerkship. If you are on a promotion or tenure granting track, your portfolio will be an important part of the information you gather to inform a very important summative evaluation, the decision whether to grant you promotion and/or tenure. Your summative evaluation should be based on a variety of observations from multiple sources.

Two important concepts govern the fairness of evaluations, and as the stakes rise in evaluation, each becomes more important. For quantitative evaluations, validity and reliability are important measures of the quality of the instrument. Validity is the extent to which the instrument measures what it purports to measure. Reliability is the degree to which the instrument reveals the same results on repeated administrations, or that multiple items within an instrument reveal similar results.

Levels of Outcomes Measured in Evaluation

Donald Kirkpatrick wrote the seminal work on evaluating training, and his levels of outcomes are often used in the education world. The four levels of outcomes for an educational intervention are listed from simplest to most complex to measure (Kirkpatrick 1977):

1. Reaction: How well did people like the educational intervention?
2. Learning: What principles, facts, techniques, ideas did they gather in the educational interaction?
3. Behavior: What changes in their performance resulted from the educational interaction?
4. Results: What was the impact of the educational interaction on the rest of the system in which the participant works?

More recently, Belfield and colleagues adapted Kirkpatrick's levels of outcomes specifically for medical education. In their adaptation, the levels are listed from most complex to simplest (Belfield et al. 2001).

1. *Healthcare outcomes:* What measurable patient/population outcomes can be demonstrated to have been changed due to the educational intervention?
2. *Health professionals' behavior, performance, or practice:* What behaviors, performance, or practices can be demonstrated to have been addressed, changed, or implemented due to the educational intervention?
3. *Learning or knowledge:* What learning or new knowledge did participants acquire in the educational intervention?
4. *Reaction or satisfaction of participants:* How well did participants like the educational intervention?
5. *Participation or completion of the educational intervention:* To what extent did people complete the intervention, or how many people completed the intervention?

Kirkpatrick notes that not all levels of outcomes will be collected for all educational interventions, and this is true of the Belfield system as well. However, in the continuing medical education world (CME), providers are expected to document the impact of the educational offerings at least at the level of showing behavior, performance, or practice change according to the new Accreditation Council for Continuing Medical Education standards. If practicing physicians are the audience for your educational interventions and you intend to offer CME credit, you will likely be expected by the accredited provider to assist them in documenting the outcomes of the educational event at that level.

Table 16.1 Outcome levels and sources for information

Belfield	Kirkpatrick	Sources	Evidence
Participation or completion		Participants	Sign in sheets, roll call, attestation of participant
Reaction or Satisfaction	Reaction	Participants, stakeholders, supervisors of participants	Written evaluation form, follow up polling of participants, follow-up requests from same audience, requests to repeat an event from a different audience, satisfaction of supervisors of audience members
Learning or Knowledge	Learning	Participants, educators who receive participants at next level	Multiple choice examination, Audience Response System quiz at end of event, follow up survey of participants, survey of "upstream" educators
Health professionals' behavior, performance or practice	Behavior	Participants, coworkers of participants, supervisors of participants	Questionnaire for participants asking about behavior, performance or practice, direct observation, interviews with others who work with providers, interviews with supervisors, focus group with participants exploring behavior, performance or practice
Healthcare outcomes	Results		Quality improvement data from healthcare organization, public health data, prescribing data from associated insurance company

Various methods can be used to gather evaluative information. Below we present a table with the Kirkpatrick and Belfield evaluation schema and suggested sources of information (Table 16.1).

Summing Up

- A teaching portfolio is a useful mechanism to document your teaching trajectory
- Part of the portfolio is your reflection on your evolution as a teacher
- Part of the portfolio is documentation of your evolution as demonstrated by your response to feedback and evaluation
- Evaluation can serve multiple purposes, including guiding your growth and providing a judgment on you or your educational interventions
- Evaluation can serve to document the outcomes of your educational interventions
- There are multiple sources you can consult for information about your teaching

References

Baldwin CD, Gusic M, Chandran L (2008) The educator portfolio: a tool for career development. Faculty Vitae. Retrieved from http://www.aamc.org/members/facultydev/facultyvitae/winter08/leadership.htm

Belfield C, Thomas H, Bullock A, Eynon R, Wall D (2001) Measuring effectiveness for best evidence medical education: a discussion. Med Teach 23(2):164–170. doi:10.1080/0142150020031084

Kirkpatrick DL (1977) Evaluation of training. In: Craig RL, Bittel LR (eds) Training and development handbook. McGraw-Hill Book Company, New York, pp 87–112

Simpson D, Fincher RM, Hafler JP, Irby DM, Richards BF, Rosenfeld GC et al (2007) Advancing educators and education by defining the components and evidence associated with educational scholarship.MedEduc41(10):1002–1009.doi:MED2844[pii]10.1111/j.1365-2923.2007.02844.x

For Further Reading

Lewis KΘ, Baker RC (2007) The development of an electronic educational portfolio: an outline for medical education professionals. Teach Learn Med 19(2):139–147

This provides a more detailed approach to developing an educational portfolio, and gives advice on how to create an electronic portfolio

Hesketh EA, Bagnall G, Buckley EG, Friedman M, Goodall E, Harden RM, Laidlaw JM, Leighton Beck I, McKinlay P, Newton R, Oughton R (2001) A framework for developing excellence as a clinical educator. Med Educ 35:555–564

The framework developed in this article serves multiple purposes, but for somebody new to medical education, it can serve to outline the various activities that medical educators undertake

Baldwin C, Chandran L, Gusic M (2011) Guidelines for evaluating the educational performance of medical school faculty: priming a national conversation. Teach Learn Med 23(3):285–297

This article elaborates how one might evaluate educator's performance, providing clear definitions of the various domains in which an educator should be evaluated. It could be used to guide the development of a portfolio that assists in documenting the trajectory of learning about teaching

Chapter 17
Teaching as Scholarship

Deborah Simpson and M. Brownell Anderson

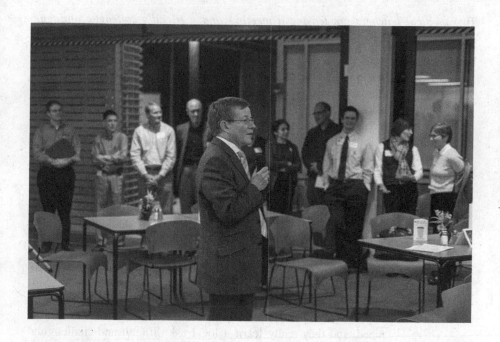

D. Simpson, Ph.D. (✉)
Department of Family Medicine at UWSMPH & MCW, Academic Affairs – Aurora Health Care, Aurora UW Medical Group/Academic Administration,
1020 North 12th Street, Suite 5120, Milwaukee, WI, USA

M.B. Anderson, M.Ed.
Senior Academic Officer, International Programs, National Board of Medical Examiners,
3750 Market Street, Philadelphia, PA 19104, USA

K.N. Huggett and W.B. Jeffries (eds.), *An Introduction to Medical Teaching*,
DOI 10.1007/978-94-017-9066-6_17, © Springer Science+Business Media Dordrecht 2014

Abstract Drawing inspiration, knowledge, support and challenges from our colleagues and from educational consultants is how we enhance teaching and learning. Similar to the need to consult with colleagues about patient care or scientific investigators, we as educators must get together and discuss our work in medical education. To achieve this shared goal, we as educators must think of ourselves as members of an educational cooperative – a teaching and learning community – where we exchange and build our collective knowledge about medical education. This chapter introduces the criteria associated with educational scholarship as teachers, curriculum developers, and authors of learner assessment tools.

Introduction

Two medical teachers are leaving a meeting and a friendly colleague dialogue begins:

Dr. Woodson: "Are you going to the visiting professor workshop on effective teaching techniques tomorrow? It's the one about teaching as a competency including adult learning principles, neurobiology of learning, and teaching strategies including simulation and digital technologies like social media."

Dr. Laszlo: "I'm not sure. I really have to get my syllabus ready by early next week."

Dr. Woodson: "Oh, I can help you with that or you could contact one of our educator consultants. I met with one last week and in less than an hour we had updated and presented my syllabus in a way that she confirmed was educationally sound and she taught me how to upload it into our learning management system. If you did that, it would give you time to come with me to the teaching workshop!"

Dr. Laszlo: "You already get good teaching ratings. Why do you want to go to this session anyway?"

Dr. Woodson: "I do get pretty good teaching ratings, but I want to continue to improve. My students tell me that I have clear goals, I am organized, and they really learn a lot. I ask difficult and challenging questions, but in a way that is non-threatening. The problem for me is, I'm not sure what I actually do; I just teach. So I really want to understand more about why what I'm doing works and about teaching competencies, simulation and social media. I've read some things by this visiting professor and his work is very informative."

Dr. Laszlo: Alright, you've convinced me to meet with an educational consultant about my course and I'll go to the workshop. I'll see you there!"

Drawing inspiration, knowledge, support and challenges from our colleagues and from educational consultants is among the ways we enhance our own teaching and learning. Similar to the need to consult with colleagues about patient care or scientific investigators, we as educators must get together and discuss our work in medical education. Teaching, like any profession, "advances when people find like-minded colleagues to work with, review their efforts and push them to the next stages of thinking" (Hutchings 2004). Yet sometimes medical teachers work in isolation. We spend significant time and effort developing course materials, lectures, syllabi, assessment tools, standardized patient cases, and evaluation forms without first seeking existing materials or colleague review of our materials.

If you are reading this chapter, it is probably because you, like Drs. Woodson and Laszlo, are dedicated to educating healthcare professionals who will provide the highest quality of care possible for their patients, their communities and their populations. To achieve this shared goal, we as educators must think of ourselves as members of an educational cooperative – a teaching and learning community – where we exchange and build our collective knowledge about medical education.

Enhancing Our Collective Knowledge About Medical Education: Adopting Educational Scholarship Criteria

Health professions educators should understand and adopt the criteria associated with educational scholarship as teachers, curriculum developers, and authors of learner assessment tools. We should seek explanations for why something works or does not work. Glassick and colleagues (1997) outlined six criteria that can guide our individual work as teachers and allow us to exchange and build our collective knowledge in health professions education.

- **Clear Goals:** The educational purpose/outcome is explicitly defined.
- **Adequate Preparation:** The teacher draws on the collective knowledge and resources in the field and has the required expertise.
- **Appropriate Methods:** The design selected including delivery strategies, tools, and approaches, is matched with the goals and best practices in the field.
- **Significant Results:** Outcomes achieved are important to the learner, educator, the program and to the field.
- **Effective Presentation:** Educator's work is shared with the community, clearly articulated and framed to build upon the collective knowledge in the field.
- **Reflective Critique:** Critical self-appraisal resulting in the identification of strengths and opportunities for improvement.

Improving as an Individual

Glassick's criteria can be reframed as guiding questions to improve our own work as educators. Consider the following:

- What are our goals as educators?
- Are we adequately prepared for our various educational roles, be it as teacher, author of a curriculum, designer of an e-learning module, advisor/mentor, peer reviewer and/or educational leader/administrator?

- What are the appropriate methods to achieve our goal(s) in each role?
- How do we know if we have achieved significant results?
- Have we presented what we learned to our colleagues in an effective way?
- Have we identified the key variables influencing our results and how to sustain and improve upon our success as part of our reflective critique?

As educators we often answer these scholarship-derived questions by reviewing student evaluations and student performance "results" to identify ways we can improve. This reflective self-critique is informed by our experiences as teachers and as learners – as demonstrated by an outstanding teacher, a key role model, or mentor. However, at some point our ability to advance our competencies as educators is limited by our own thinking, leading to the recognition that we are inadequately prepared! It is at that point we must seek out other resources, drawing on the knowledge available in the field of education as a means to achieve our goals, expand our methods, perhaps reinforce our findings, and/or improve the effective presentation of our results.

Dr. Woodson is the perfect example of an educator who has recognized the need for adequate preparation. While students rate her teaching highly, Dr. Woodson is unable to explain why what she does as a teacher is valued by her students. Therefore Dr. Woodson seeks to enhance her preparation by drawing upon the collective knowledge in the field. Attendance at the workshop is an appropriate method to achieve her goals, but there are a variety of effective methods that draw upon the available knowledge base.

- Read books like this, reference materials, articles in journals on medical education and teaching.
- Talk to colleagues who are excellent teachers and ask them how they improve, what they would do in this situation, invite them to review materials and observe our teaching.
- Attend (face-to-face or online) educational workshops to learn how to write objectives, design assessment materials, and/or critique literature in the field.
- Critically reflect about a difficult teaching experience. This can range from an informal analysis to the more formal process of recording a critical incident and forcing oneself to step back and think about what worked, what didn't work and why. Share this with a colleague and get their feedback.
- Seek input from learners, asking them what worked, what didn't work and how to improve, both through informal mechanisms (e.g., at the end of a session), or through formal mechanisms (e.g., online questionnaires and surveys).
- Use the worksheets in the AAMC Toolbox for Evaluating Educators to affirm that your teaching, curriculum, and/or assessment tools have fulfilled Glassick's scholarship criteria and revise as needed (Gusic et al. 2013).
- Enroll in a faculty development program, medical education fellowship, certificate program, or formal degree program to continue to build and expand your knowledge about medical education, improve specific educator competencies and/or explore collaborative opportunities.

- Attend medical education meetings through your professional organizations or the larger community of medical educators regionally to globally to learn about new strategies, techniques and resources in the field.

Replenishing and Enhancing Our Collective Knowledge About Health Professions Education

As an individual, Dr. Woodson can draw on the knowledge available in the field to achieve her teaching improvement goals. However, when we as medical educators only draw from the knowledge and resources in our cooperative community, we ultimately drain our collective knowledge reservoir. Our collective knowledge must be continuously replenished or, like a river from which water is drawn to grow crops, it will eventually stagnate and run dry.

In order to replenish and enrich our fund of educational knowledge, we as medical educators must actively contribute to our collective knowledge about what works, what doesn't work, and why. Again, Glassick's scholarship criteria can be used to determine the value of contributions to our collective knowledge. Does the contribution have clear goals? Was it prepared building on what we already know? Were appropriate methods utilized in its design, development, delivery, assessment, and/or evaluation? Were the results significant? Is the contribution effectively presented so that it can be understood and used by members of our cooperative community of educators? Does it include an assessment of strengths, weaknesses and opportunities?

To achieve the shared goal of preparing health professionals to provide the highest quality of care, as educators we must move from isolation (e.g., giving lectures, presentations, designing curriculum and assessment tools) to engagement with the educational community (drawing resources from and contributing to our collective knowledge). In 2006, the *Association of American Medical Colleges-Group on Educational Affairs* sponsored a consensus conference on educational scholarship. Building on over 15 years of work in defining the attributes of educational scholarship, the Q^2 Engage model emerged (Simpson et al. 2007). This model emphasized the need to transition from isolation as a teacher to engagement in a community of educators. Academies of educators have been established at our health professions colleges and universities, teaching hospitals, and our professional societies to help engage educators in systematically advancing educators and education (Searle et al. 2010; LaMantia et al. 2012). This engagement begins by drawing resources from and, as appropriate, contributing resources to the collected knowledge about how best to teach, assess, and evaluate our learners and programs toward the goal of outstanding patient, community and population based healthcare.

Let's return to the examples of our two colleagues that began this chapter and use that conversation to highlight how faculty can naturally engage with the community of medical educators consistent with Glassick's scholarship criteria.

Replenishing and Enhancing the Collective Knowledge Through Engagement

Dr. Woodson, who sought to understand *why* she is an effective teacher, did indeed attend the teaching workshop by the visiting professor; gaining a new understanding of how students learn and instructional technology strategies. Armed with this new knowledge, Dr. Woodson then expanded her teaching strategies and skills, sought feedback from students and colleagues about her teaching, reflected on the results and revised her goals.

This continuous cycle, starting with Dr. Woodson's clear goal of teaching improvement, to adequate preparation via readings, workshop attendance, discussions with colleagues, through reflective critique demonstrates the use of Glassick's scholarship criteria. This process can also be used to guide an educator's step-wise development of instruction, a learner assessment tool, or a program evaluation instrument, beginning as always with a clear goal and adequate preparation by drawing on what is known in the field (Gusic et al. 2013).

Contributing to Collective Knowledge Through Consultation and Presentations

For Dr. Woodson, her teaching successes resulted in several teaching awards both within her department and at the school-wide level. Over time, colleagues began asking Dr. Woodson for guidance about how to improve their teaching. She co-taught a local workshop on effective teaching and then organized the workshop materials and results into a faculty development module accepted by MedEdPORTAL following peer review. Dr. Woodson was invited to serve as a visiting education professor in her specialty at another medical school.

During her visiting professor presentation, Dr. Woodson acknowledged the lack of significant results specific to effective teaching in her own specialty. On the way back from her visiting professorship, Dr. Woodson reflected on the audience's questions and realized that they highlighted the need for specialty-specific teaching effectiveness knowledge. Back at work, Dr. Woodson talked to several of her colleagues about this need with an emphasis on clear goals, adequate preparation as teachers, and appropriate teaching methods.

Inquiry into a Gap in Our Collective Knowledge

Through her *effective analysis* of the gaps in our understanding about specialty-specific effective teaching and the Q & A results from her visiting professor lectureship, Dr. Woodson engaged her specialty colleagues, her school's librarian and the school's educator consultant to help her address these gaps. The consultant guided Dr. Woodson and the team through the selection of *appropriate methods* to yield the *results* that would answer their questions. The inquiry team then worked on how to *effectively present* and contribute the results to the broader educational community. Upon reflection, Dr. Woodson realized that contributing to the medical education knowledge reservoir was professionally stimulating and merely required engagement with her educator colleague community using the scholarship criteria in a step wise progression beginning with clear goals.

Engaging with Your Colleagues to Address Gaps in Our Collective Knowledge

As practicing health professions teachers who seek excellence in education, questions and curiosities about the teaching and learning process emerge on a daily basis. Almost all the questions begin with "Why", "How" or "What." For example:

- Why did my (small group, clinical, lab) teaching work so well last month but not with this month's students?
- Why is the (OSCE, quiz, licensure exam) performance going up/down when we are teaching the same core content as last year?
- Why don't our students ever talk with patients and address health risk situations/behaviors (e.g., obesity, violence, smoking, unprotected sex, alcoholism/drug abuse – name your topic)?
- How can I improve my course? Module? Program?
- How can I get more students interested in caring for patients who are (geriatric, impoverished, abused) or who have chronic illnesses (diabetes, hypertension, asthma)?
- What would happen if I just stopped lecturing and put everything online and used social media?

As soon as you begin to explore your questions you are engaged with your educational community through reading the literature, talking with colleagues, attending workshops, and/or seeking consultations. By drawing on the knowledge in our field you can at least partially answer your questions and you will naturally begin to identify the gaps in what we know and consider ways to fill those gaps. Once you have effectively presented the results that fill a gap, you have contributed to our collective knowledge.

It is through this process of engagement – beginning with the question(s) that emerge through your daily work as a teacher and then drawing from and contributing to our collective knowledge about education – that medical educators can advance as individual teachers and advance the field of health professions education. Clear goals, adequate preparation, appropriate methods, significant results, effective presentation and reflective critique are the hallmarks of this engagement process (see Table 17.1).

Table 17.1 Engagement with community of educators – Dr. Woodson's example

Focus of activity →	Engagement with collective knowledge in our field	
Glassick's criteria ↓	Individual – *Draws from*	Community of Educators – *Contributes to*
Clear goals	Understand and improve own teaching effectiveness	Improve others teaching effectiveness (colleague questions)
	Assess your educator competencies, identify gaps, set goals	Answer question/gap in collective knowledge regarding specialty-specific teaching effectiveness
Adequate preparation	Read literature	Continue to learn about effective teaching (e.g., read)
	Talk with colleagues	Give informal guidance to colleagues in response to requests
	Attend (listen to) visiting professor workshop(s)	Give presentations on effective teaching
	Enroll in education program	
	Join an education learning community/academy	
Appropriate methods	Try new teaching strategies/ approaches	Listen to audience questions
	Ask for feedback from learners	Form a collaborative group with needed expertise to explore questions
Significant results	Review results including student feedback, learning performance measures relative to goals	Addresses a gap in collective knowledge related to specialty-specific teaching
Effective presentation	Display your results in a form that is available for colleagues to review, critique and provide input	Share those results in a form that others can understand and build from
Reflective critique	Evaluate strengths/weaknesses and define specific goals for continued improvement	Reflect on audience questions to identify gap → new goal based on recognition of gap in collective knowledge

Effectively Presenting Teaching as Scholarship: Adapting to Audience

What if this chapter had begun by advising you that your advancement and recognition as a teacher depends on your ability to identify an important question, design a study to answer that question, and publish the study results? Would that introduction have motivated you to "publish"? Would that introduction connect with your goals and motivations as a teacher? Effective teachers achieve their objectives by adapting their teaching approach to their learners' needs, goals and ambitions.

Our experience is that all teachers want to provide outstanding educational experiences for their learners so that their learners will, in turn, provide the highest quality of health care possible for patients, communities and populations. However, when the emphasis is on "publishing" and "scholarship" the dynamic relationship between "teaching," "learning," and "scholarship" is often lost. Designing and delivering instruction, like medicine, must be an evidence-based performance art. To excel as teachers we must draw from the best practices and resources in our field, and as professionals we understand the need to give back, adding to the collective knowledge in our field. Applying the Glassick criteria to our work as teachers provides a common framework making the relationship between our daily work as teachers and our contributions to the field transparent.

You may well be asking, "How do I begin?" Start with

- **Clear goals:** What do you care about as a teacher? Do you have any "Why…, How…, What…, Questions"? Talk to a colleague to help you refine and clarify your goal.
- **Adequate preparation:** Read about it. Talk to colleagues. Attend a workshop or meeting on that topic. If you are interested in more information about teaching as scholarship, and how to document your work as a teacher, see the resources listed in Guided Reading.
- **Appropriate methodology:** Based on this preparation select an appropriate approach and try it.
- **Significant results:** Seek to determine if your approach worked! Engage your learners in this new approach by asking for their feedback and evaluation. Examine the data on your learners' performance, satisfaction and motivation. In addition to survey data, there are other indicators of effective teaching. For example, do your learners now arrive prepared? Are they early or on time (rather than late)? Do they remain active and alert throughout your session? If the performance data are the same but your learners' report that your teaching strategy was more effective, is that a significant result?
- **Effective presentation:** Who else would be interested in what you have learned? Was this a question/problem of local interest only? You could address this by talking to your colleagues, holding a conference, sending a brief email, and/or reporting at a faculty meeting. If this was a "gap" in our collective knowledge in the field (e.g., the literature, peer reviewed educational repositories) then tell us about it in a way that we can understand, use, and build on! As teachers, effective presentation should be our strength as we constantly adapt our teaching to effectively communicate with different learners. Presenting our work to colleagues is merely another form of adapting to your learners!
- **Reflective critique:** Self-assessment is a critical skill and one that should be done individually and with peers. Use the knowledge gained through your adequate preparation, selection of methods, results, and presentation to identify what worked, what did not work and next steps. And as you might guess this step provides you with "clear goals" for your continued teaching, learning, scholarship and engagement with other educators.

Reprise:
To demonstrate this dynamic relationship let us pay a return visit, several years later to Drs. Woodson and Laszlo:

Dr. Laszlo: "Dr. Woodson, congratulations on your election as president of our Teaching Academy! Your leadership will help us build new forums and expand on our established sessions for bringing educators together to critically discuss how our students' learn and how we teach."

Dr. Woodson: "Thank you, it is indeed an honor. And I am glad to see that you are so active in our academy as well. I hope I can count on you to lead some of our sessions. I remember a couple of years ago when I had to convince you to go to our visiting medical education professor session."

Dr. Laszlo: "Indeed, your encouragement and nudging got me out of my office to work with others on education. I had always felt like I had to do it myself or I was somehow not fulfilling my roles and responsibilities as a teacher. Talking and learning from other educators has really improved my teaching and I even have some competency-based instructional materials and assessment tools published in one of the peer reviewed repositories."

Dr. Woodson: "That's fabulous, congratulations! It often just takes some encouragement from our colleagues to prompt us to participate in the process of drawing from and contributing to our educational community. So can I encourage you again? Would you lead our education journal club for the next year?"

Dr. Laszlo: I'd be delighted to serve as the education journal club convener. It would allow me to expand the "Educator Reading Club" – part of our residency's medical education fellowship track– to include students and faculty.

Dr. Woodson: "What a great idea! Are there some students or residents who could help as co-conveners?"

Dr. Laszlo: "Yes indeed! One of the residents in our medical education track would be ideal to help pull this group together… Ah, here he is now. Dr. Woodson, please let me introduce you to Dr. Matthew Scott. Dr. Scott is a wonderful teacher and his students are always telling me about how Dr. Scott's golf analogies help them really understand…"

References

Glassick CE, Hubert MT, Maeroff GI (1997) Scholarship assessed: evaluation of the professoriate. Jossey-Bass, San Francisco

Gusic M, Amiel J, Baldwin C, Chandran L, Fincher R, Mavis B, O'Sullivan P, Padmore J, Rose S, Simpson D, Strobel H, Timm C, Viggiano T (2013) Using the AAMC Toolbox for Evaluating Educators: You be the Judge!. MedEdPORTAL; 2013. Cited 23 April 2013, Available from: www.mededportal.org/publication/9313

Hutchings P (2004) Building a better conversation about learning. Carnegie perspectives. The Carnegie Foundation for the Advancement of Teaching. Cited 23 April 2013. Available via http://www.carnegiefoundation.org/perspectives/sub.asp?key=245&subkey=582

LaMantia J, Hamstra SJ, Martin DR, Searle N et al (2012) Faculty development in medical education research. Acad Emerg Med 19:1462–1467

Searle N, Thompson B, Friedland J et al (2010) The prevalence and practice of academies of medical education: a survey of U.S. medical schools. Acad Med 85:48–56

Simpson D, Fincher RM, Hafler JP, Irby DM, Richards BF, Rosenfeld GC, Viggiano TR (2007) Advancing educators and education by defining the components and evidence associated with educational scholarship. Med Educ 41(10):1002–1009

For Further Reading

Ferguson KJ, Wolter EM, Yarbrough DB, Carline JD, Krupat E (2009) Defining and describing medical learning communities: results of a national survey. Acad Med 84(11):1549–1556

Ferguson et al., identify the most important features of the learning communities based on a literature review and survey of academic deans of all U.S. and Canadian medical schools (N=124) to identify existing learning communities (N=18)

Hafler JP, Morzinski JA, Blanco MA, Fincher RME (2012) Chapter 24: Educational scholarship. In: Morgenstern BZ, Alliance for Clinical Education (eds) Guidebook for clerkship directors, 4th edn. Gegensatz Press, North Syracuse. Cited 23 April 2013

Written for physicians who direct clinical clerkships/rotations for medical students, this easy to read chapter provides a brief historical perspective on educational scholarship and outlines it key elements with examples

Hodges BD, Lingard L (eds) (2012) The question of competence. Cornell University Press, Ithaca

Competency-based education is ubiquitous in health professions education. While a comprehensive literature review on competence – from definitions to assessment – is provided, the book's power lay in reminding us to question the underlying assumptions associated with competence. As the editors/authors examine competency through an array of lenses including teamwork, emotion competence, expertise, and self-assessment – you will learn and find ideas to think and talk with colleagues about for a long time to come

O'Sullivan PS, Irby DM (2011) Reframing research on faculty development. Acad Med 86(4):421–428

In support of establishing networks of educator learning communities, these distinguished authors advocate for advancing research on faculty development in medical education by learning from research in related fields such as teacher education, continuing medical education and workplace learning. The authors identify two communities of practice: the community created among participants in faculty development programs and the communities of teaching practice in the workplace (classroom or clinic) where teaching actually occurs. They identify key components of faculty development (professional development) and the environment in which faculty work and teach

Srinivasan M, Li ST, Meyers FJ, Pratt DD et al (2011) "Teaching as a Competency": competencies for medical educators. Acad Med 86(10):1211–1220

Uses the ACGME competencies and the CanMeds model to frame specific educator competencies (program design/implementation; evaluation/scholarship; leadership, mentorship) and define critical skills based on four core values (learner engagement, learner-centeredness, adaptability, self-reflection)

Shulman LS (1993) Teaching as community property: putting an end to pedagogical solitude. Change 25(6):6–7

As President of the Carnegie Foundation for the Advancement of Teaching, Dr. Lee Shulman articulated the need to make what we do as educators' public, available for peer review, and accessible in a form that others can build upon, so that education becomes "community property." Dr. Shulman's work, and that of his Carnegie colleagues (Drs. Mary Huber, Pat Hutchings, Eugene Glassick, Molly Cooke, David Irby, et al.) are informative and delightful reads guaranteed to promote reflection, clarity of goals, and remind all of us that we have an obligation as teachers to share and exchange our work. Original essays and book citations including the recent series on preparation for the professions (including medicine, nursing, clergy, law) are available under resources/publications on the foundation's website http://www.carnegiefoundation.org/. Cited 23 April 2013

Appendix

Additional Information About Medical Education

As your journey into medical education unfolds, you may want to refer to advanced resources in the field. Below we have compiled a list of medical education resources that should help your teaching career.

Medical Education Publications

Academic Medicine: This is the official journal of the Association of American Medical Colleges (AAMC). This journal publishes articles pertaining to the organization and operation of academic medical centers, emerging themes and contemporary issues and medical education research findings. http://journals.lww.com/academicmedicine

Advances in Health Sciences Education: This journal is a forum for scholarly and state-of-the art research into all aspects of health sciences education. http://www.springer.com/education+%26+language/journal/10459

British Medical Journal: The British Medical Journal publishes a series of articles entitled "ABC of Teaching and Learning in Medicine." The series covers various practical aspects of medical education. http://www.bmj.com

The Clinical Teacher: This is a publication of the Association for the Study of Medical Education. Designed for clinicians who teach, this journal aims to provide "easy access to the latest research, practice and thinking in medical education presented in a readable, stimulating and practical style." http://www.theclinicalteacher.com

Focus on Health Professional Education: This is a refereed journal sponsored by the Association for Health Professional Education It is primarily directed at educators and students in the Western Pacific Region of Australia, New Zealand, and South-East Asia. www.anzahpe.org

K.N. Huggett and W.B. Jeffries (eds.), *An Introduction to Medical Teaching,*
DOI 10.1007/978-94-017-9066-6, © Springer Science+Business Media Dordrecht 2014

Journal of the American Medical Association: This journal publishes an annual issue devoted to articles on medical education. http://jama.ama-assn.org

Medical Science Educator: Medical Science Educator is the successor of the journal *JIAMSE* and is a peer-reviewed publication of the International Association of Medical Science Educators (IAMSE). This electronic journal publishes original research, reviews, editorials and opinion papers on medical education. http://www.medicalscienceeducator.org/

Journal of Interprofessional Care: This journal publishes original, peer reviewed papers of interest to those working on collaboration in education, practice and research between medicine, nursing, allied health, veterinary science and other health related fields. http://informahealthcare.com/journal/jic

Medical Education: This journal is published by the Association for the Study of Medical Education (ASME). Medical Education is a prominent journal in the field of education for health care professionals, and primarily publishes research related to undergraduate education, postgraduate training, continuing professional development and interprofessional education. http://www.mededuc.com

Medical Education Online: This is an online journal that publishes peer-reviewed investigations in medical education. http://www.med-ed-online.org

Medical Teacher: This journal is published by the Association for Medical Education in Europe (AMEE). Medical Teacher offers descriptions of new teaching methods, guidance on structuring courses and assessing achievement, and is a forum for communication between medical teachers and those involved in general education. http://www.medicalteacher.org/

New England Journal of Medicine: This top clinical journal also publishes occasional articles devoted to the topic of medical education. http://www.nejm.org/

Teaching and Learning in Medicine: This is an international forum for scholarly research on medical teaching and assessment. The journal addresses practical issues and provides the analysis and empirical research needed to facilitate decision making about medical education. http://www.siumed.edu/dme/TLM.html

Understanding Medical Education: This is a series of extended papers produced by ASME that addresses special topics in medical education. http://www.asme.org.uk/shop/understanding-medical-education.html?maxproduct=12

Curriculum Resources and Repositories

Best Evidence in Medical Education (BEME): BEME is an international group devoted to dissemination of information about the best practices in medical education. They produce useful systematic reviews that reflect the best evidence available for various topics. http://www.bemecollaboration.org

Multimedia Educational Resource for Learning and Online Teaching (MERLOT): MERLOT is a free searchable collection of peer reviewed and selected online learning materials. This collection contains materials from all fields, but does feature a large repository of health sciences content. Resources are available for use under terms described by the author and users may also contribute content to the repository as well. http://www.merlot.org

MedEdPORTAL: MedEdPORTAL is a free publishing venue and dissemination portal sponsored by the Association of American Medical Colleges. It features peer reviewed online teaching and learning resources in medical and health professions education including tutorials, virtual patients, cases, lab manuals, assessment instruments, and faculty development materials. MedEdPORTAL covers undergraduate, graduate, and continuing medical education. Users can also contribute materials for peer review and publication. http://www.aamc.org/mededportal

Health Education Assets Library (HEAL): HEAL is a digital library of peer reviewed multimedia teaching resources for the health sciences. HEAL provides access to tens of thousands of images, videoclips, animations, presentations, and audio files that support healthcare education. Users can contribute media files for inclusion into the library. http://library.med.utah.edu/heal/

Organizations

In addition to publishing scholarly journals medical education organizations offer many other benefits, especially the opportunity to interact and network with medical teachers and scholars. The following organizations offer a variety of venues for faculty development and scholarship of teaching such as annual meetings, special conferences, online faculty development opportunities, etc.

Association for Medical Education in Europe (AMEE): The Association for Medical Education in Europe is a worldwide organization including teachers, researchers, administrators, curriculum developers, assessors and students in medicine and the healthcare professions. AMEE hosts an annual meeting and offers courses on teaching, assessment and research skills for teachers in the healthcare professions. http://www.amee.org

Association for the Study of Medical Education (ASME): ASME "seeks to improve the quality of medical education by bringing together individuals and organizations with interests and responsibilities in medical and healthcare education." www.asme.org.uk

Association of American Medical Colleges (AAMC): The AAMC is an organization of allopathic medical schools in the United States and Canada. The AAMC hosts meetings that deal with topics of interest to all aspects of medical education: organizational issues, research and best practices in medical education, student affairs and postgraduate training. The Group on Educational Affairs of the AAMC also hosts regional conferences devoted to curriculum and medical education research. www.aamc.org

Australian and New Zealand Association for Health Professional Educators (ANZAHPE): ANZAHPE is an organization that promotes education in the health professions and fosters research, continuing education, and communication between educators in the health professions. AZAME's scope includes undergraduate and postgraduate training and continuing education. www.anzahpe.org

International Association of Medical Science Educators (IAMSE): IAMSE follows the guiding principle that "all who teach the sciences fundamental to medical practice should have access to the most current information and skills needed to excel as educators." IAMSE sponsors an annual meeting as well as other conferences and faculty development activities and publishes a journal. http://iamse.org/

International Ottawa Conferences on Medical Education: This biennial conference is held alternately in North America and elsewhere in the world. This conference focuses on development of education in the healthcare professions by providing a forum for the discussion, debate and the reporting of innovations in the field of assessment. http://www.ottawaconference.org

Panamerican Federation of Associations of Medical Schools (PAFAMS): PAFAMS is a private, non-profit, non-governmental organization whose mission is the promotion and advancement of medical education and the biomedical sciences in the American Continent. http://www.fepafempafams.org/

World Federation for Medical Education (WFME): The WFME is a global organization representing six regional associations for medical education. It is primarily concerned with enhancement of the quality of medical education worldwide through establishment of standards. http://www.wfme.org/

Index

Printed in the United States
By Bookmasters